The Miracle of Acupuncture

FOREIGN LANGUAGES PRESS BEIJING

First edition 1993

ISBN 0-8351-2926-8
ISBN 7-119-01530-3

Published by Foreign Languages Press
24 Baiwanzhuang Road, Beijing 100037, China

Printed by Beijing Foreign Languages Printing House
19 Chegongzhuang Xilu, Beijing 100044, China

Distributed by China International Book Trading Corporation
35 Chegongzhuang Xilu, Beijing 100044, China
P.O. Box 399, Beijing, China

Printed in the People's Republic of China

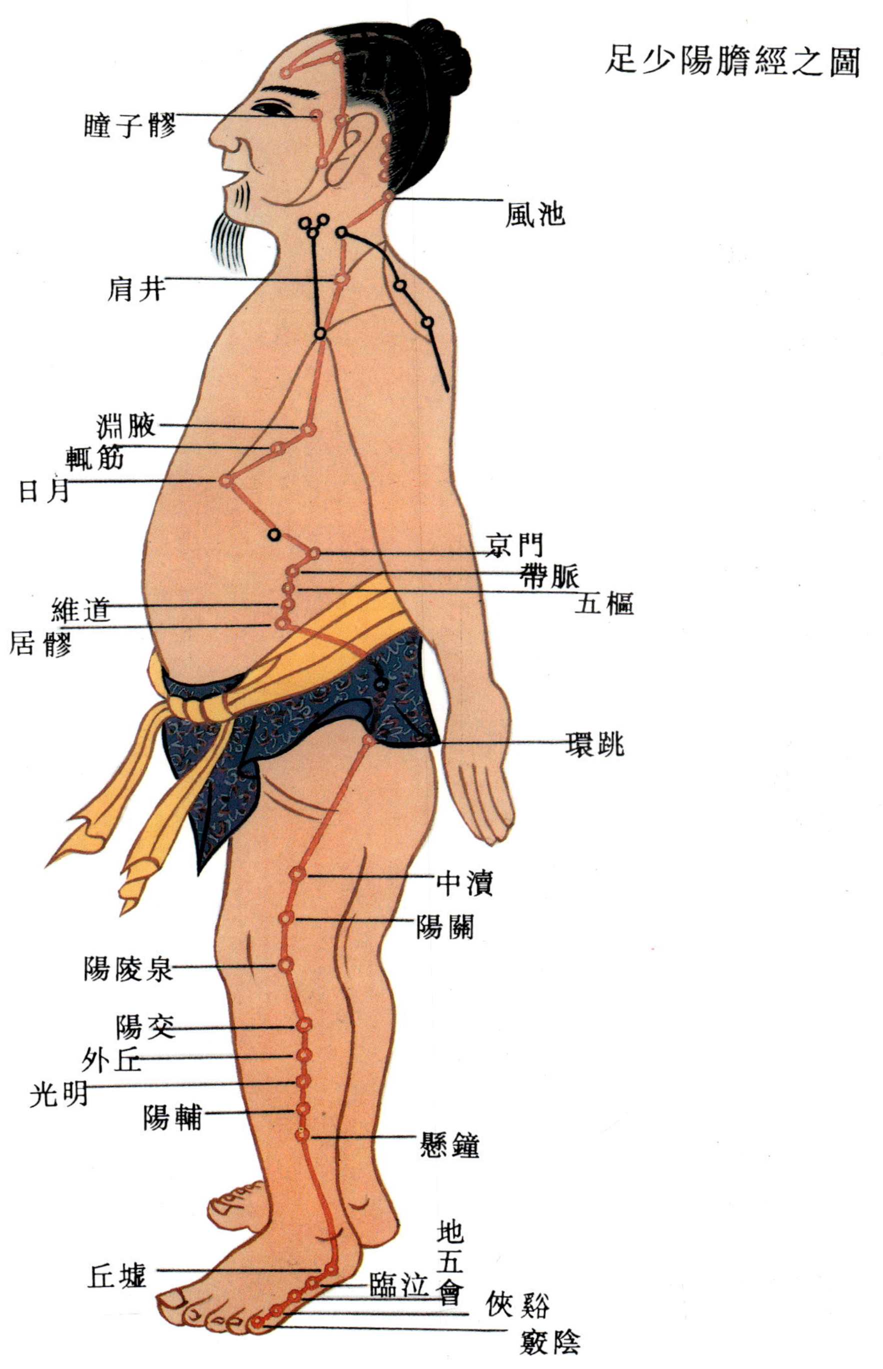

Fig. 1 The Gallbladder Meridian of Foot-*shaoyang*.

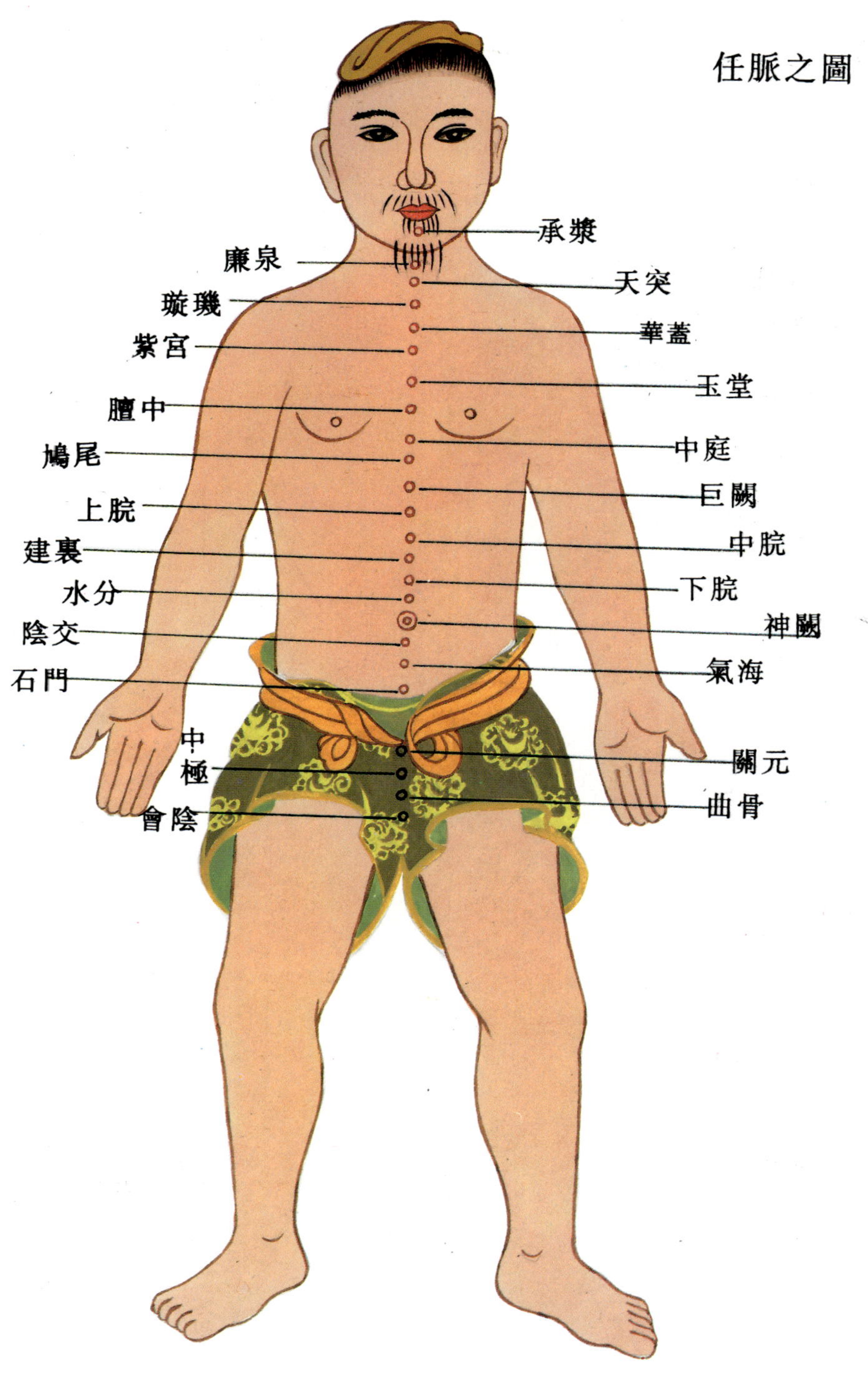

Fig. 2 The Ren Meridian.

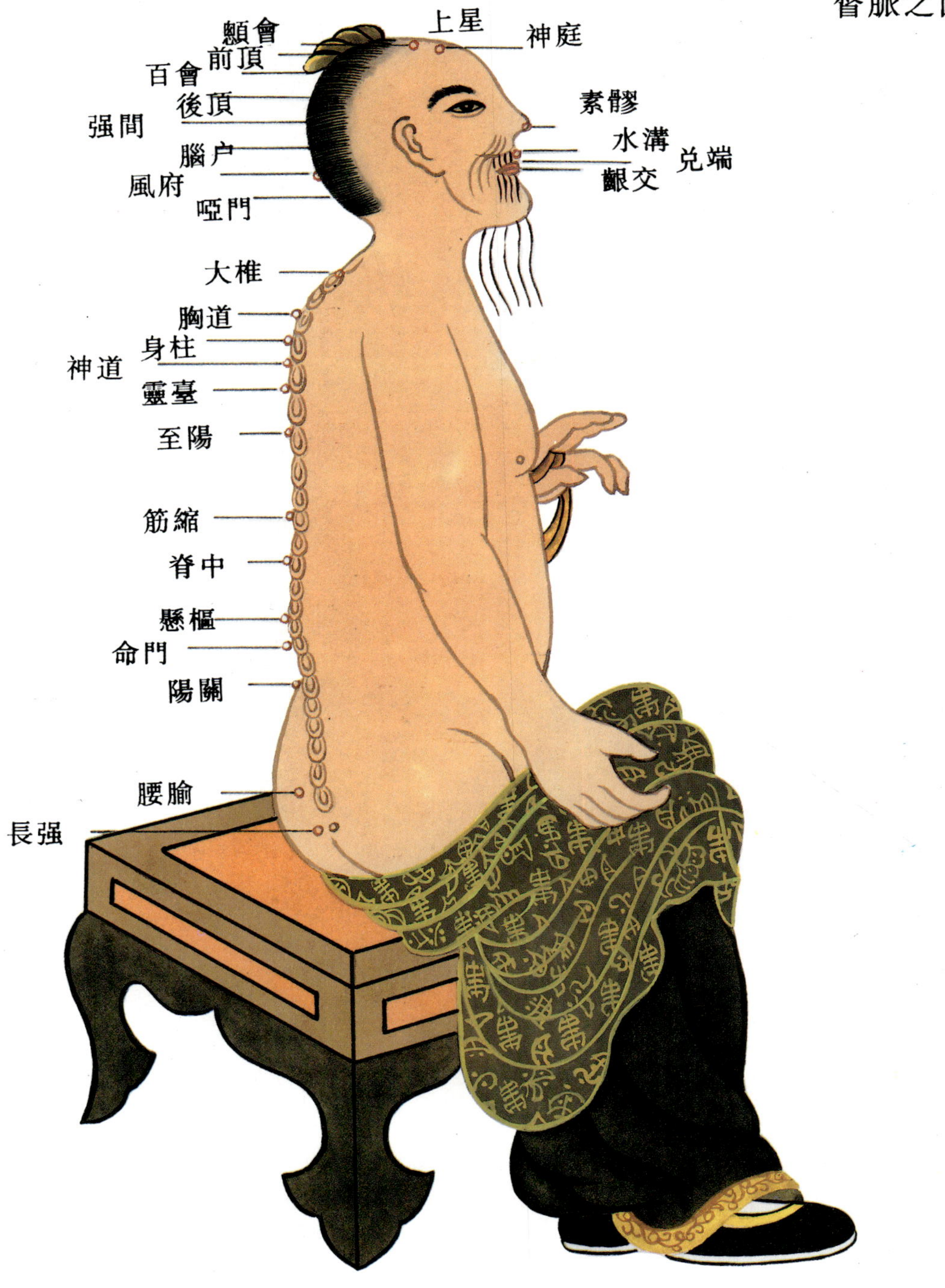

Fig. 3 The Du Meridian.

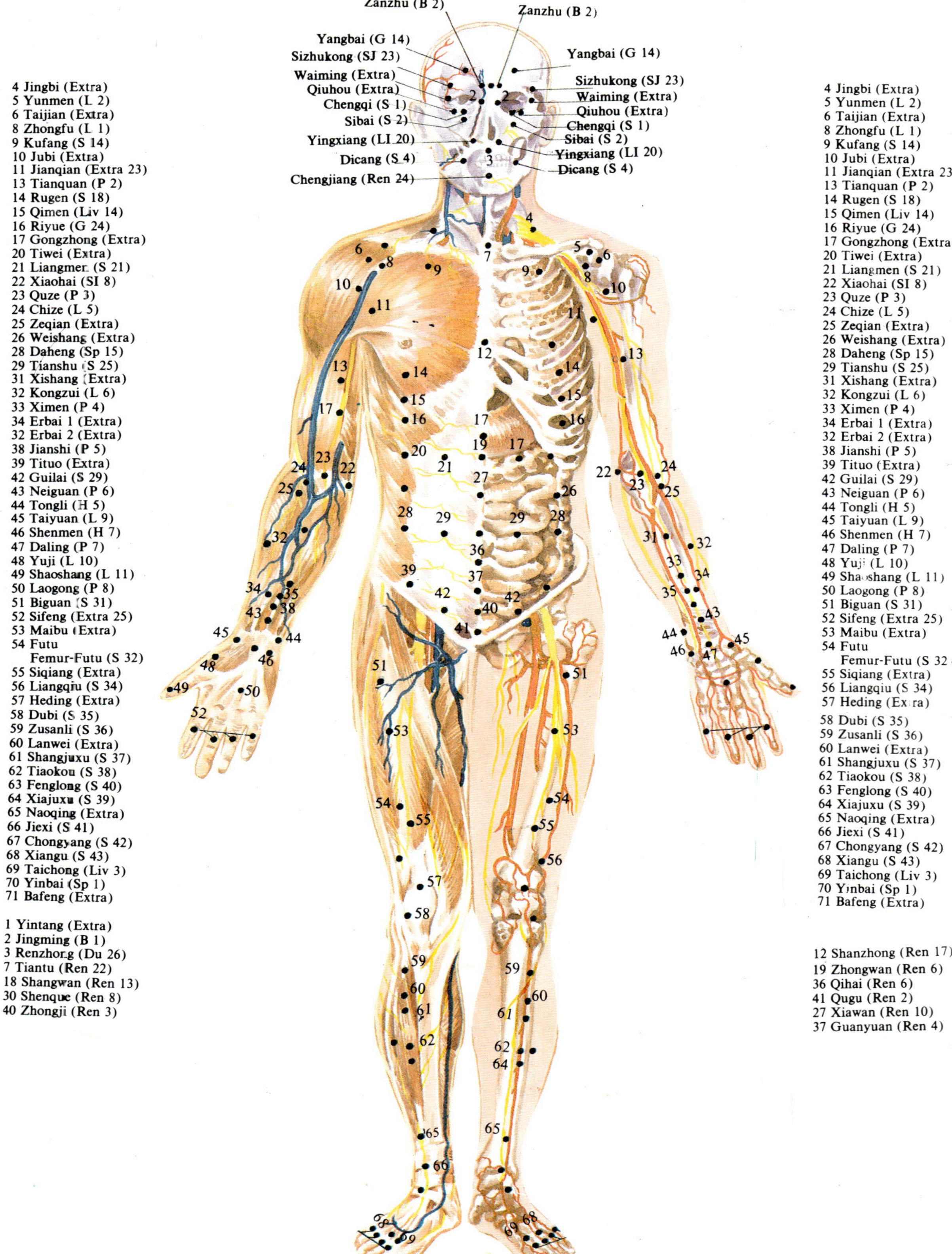

Fig. 4 Anterior Acupuncture Points

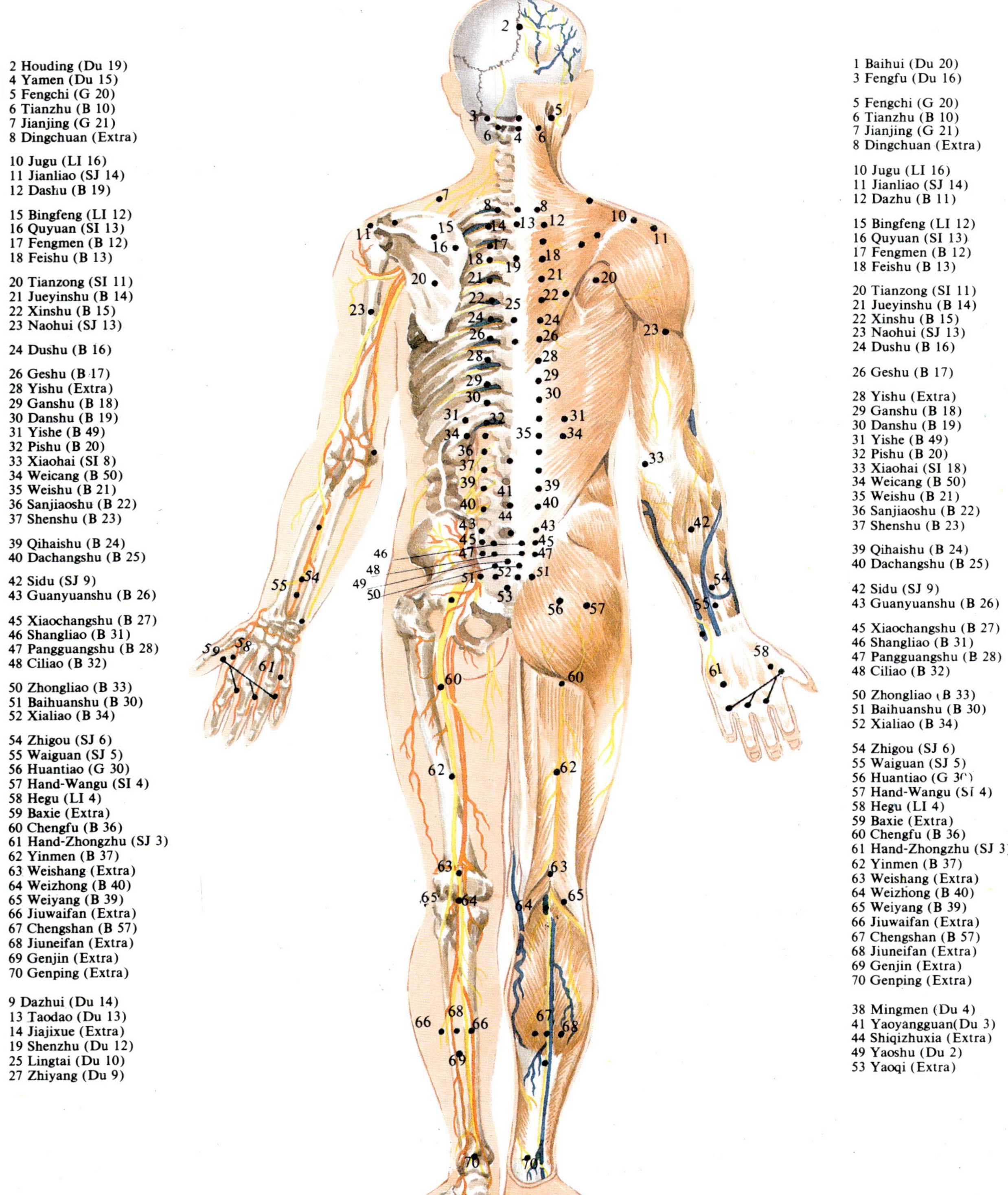

Fig. 5 Posterior Acupuncture Points

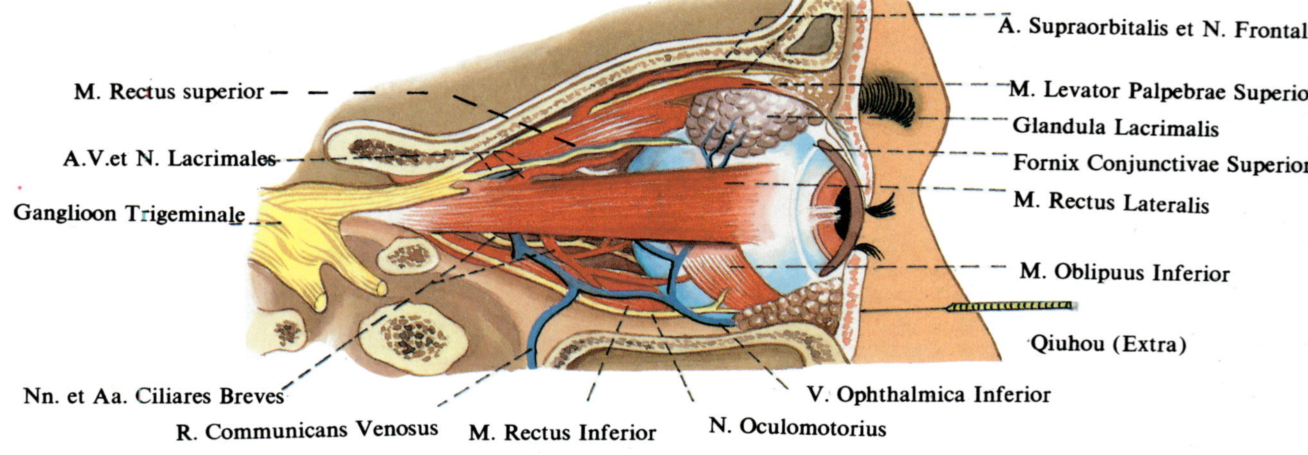

The relationship between the needle insertion direction at the *Qiuhou* acupoint and the anatomical structure of the ocular region.

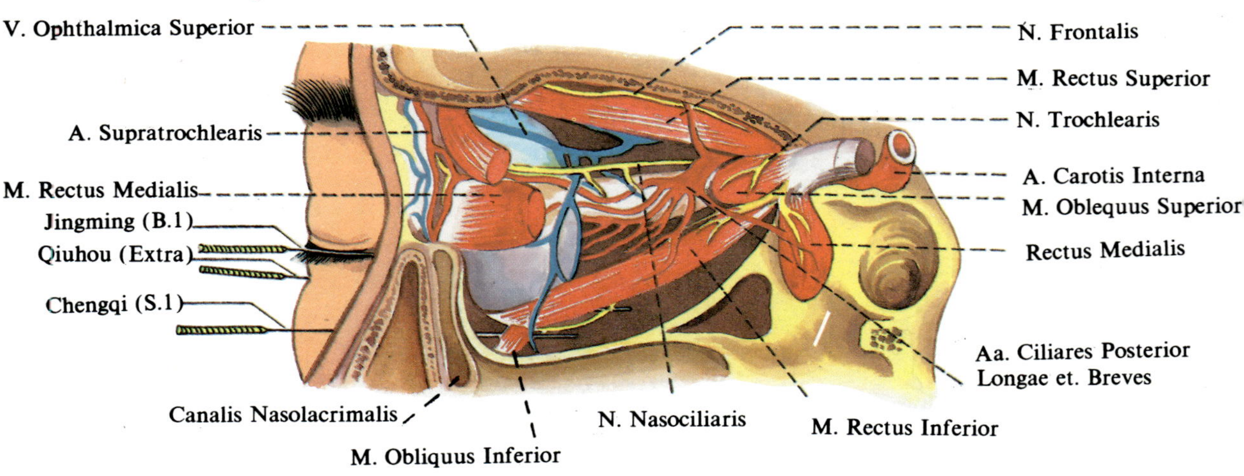

Fig. 6 Another view of the anatomical structure of the ocular region showing needle insertion directions for several acupoints.

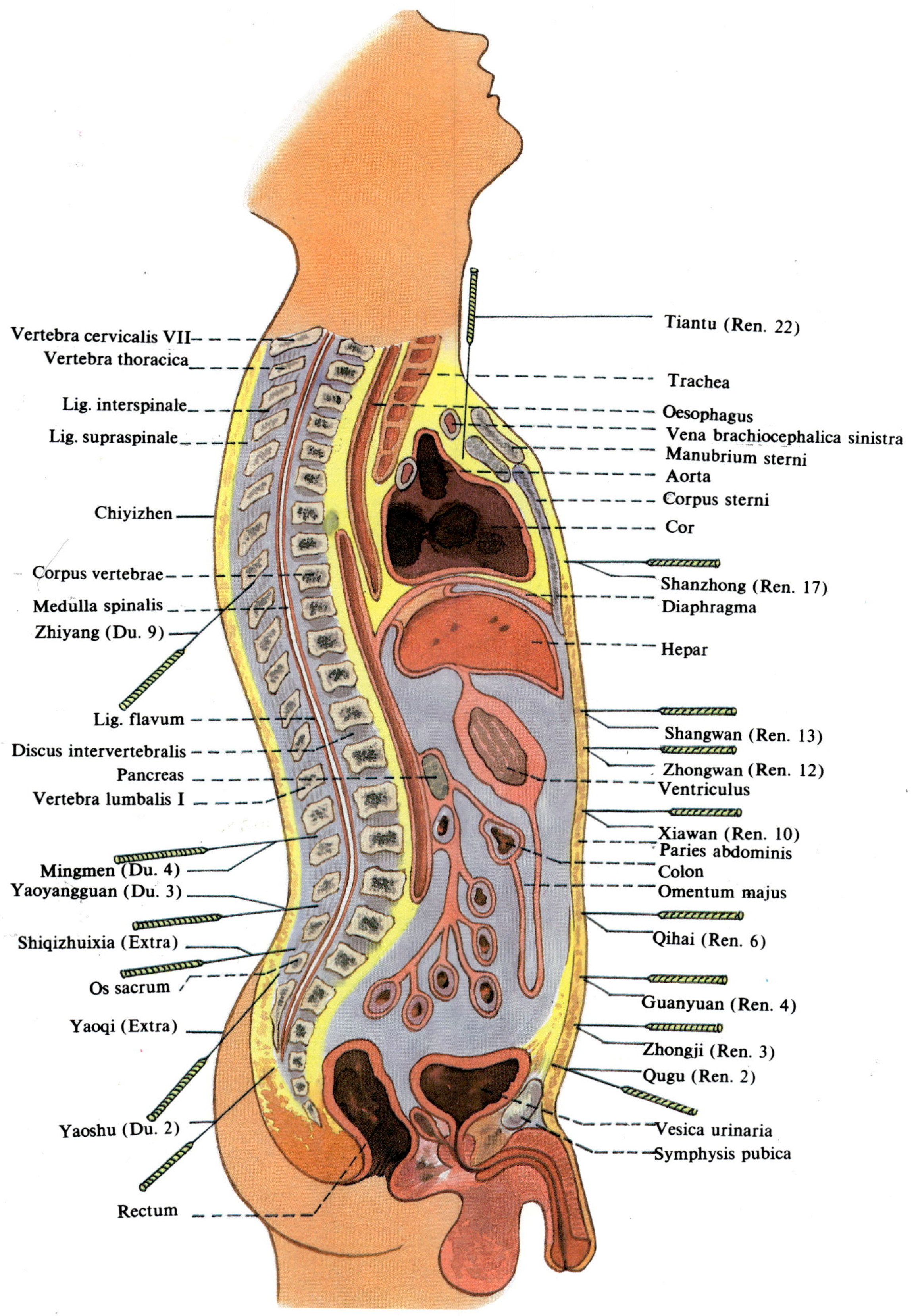

Fig. 7 The relationship between several acupoints and the anatomical structure of the sagittal cross section of the trunk.

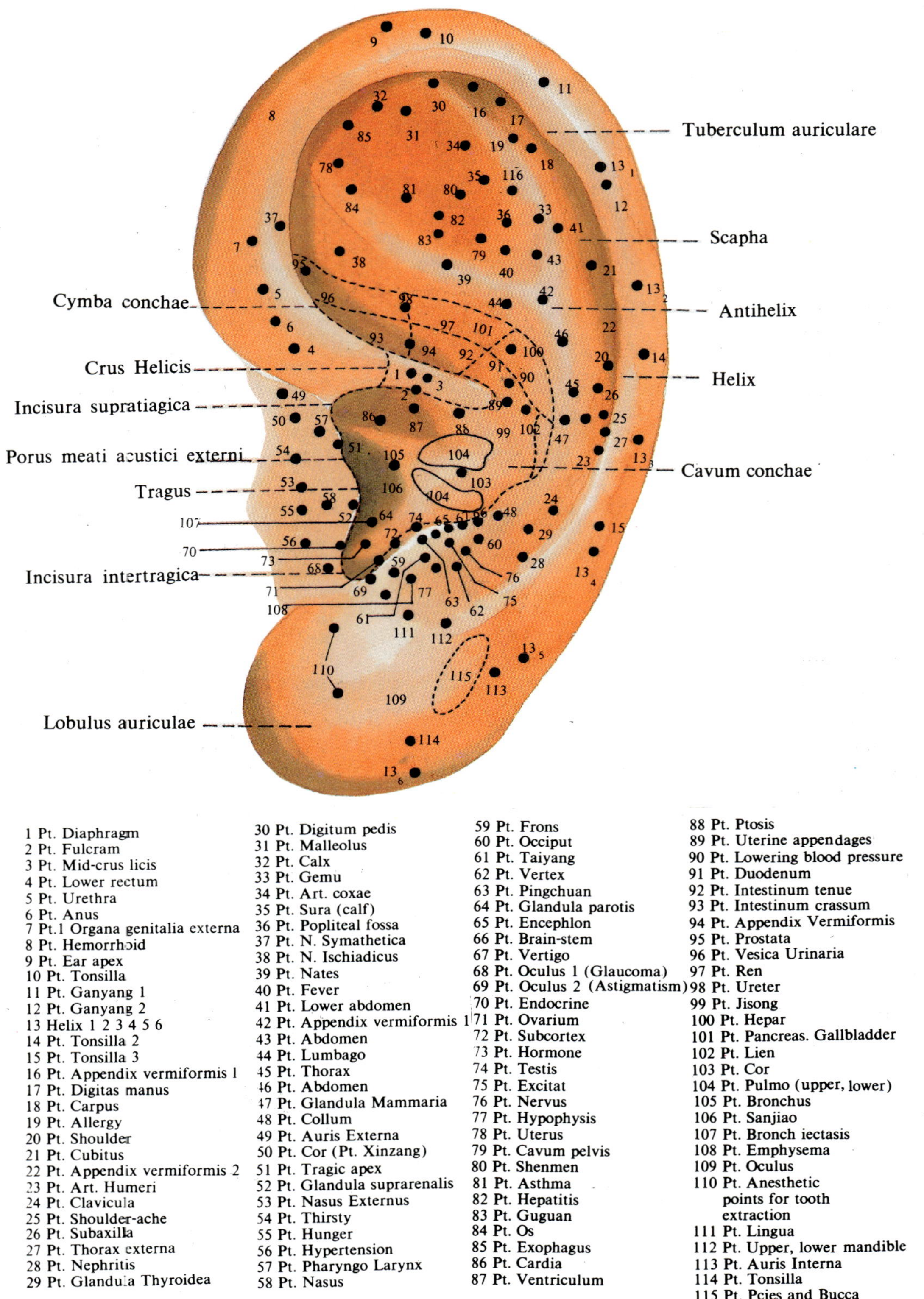

Fig. 8 The relationship between the acupoints and the superficial anatomical structure of the left auricle.

Contents

Chapter I
An Outline of the Treatment

The therapy of acupuncture and moxibustion is to stimulate a certain point on the human body with metallic needles and moxa, activating the meridians and collaterals and regulating the function of the internal organs, qi and blood, so as to prevent and treat disease. Therefore, the student must know not only the meridians, collaterals, points and manipulations but also the essentials of traditional Chinese medicine. Clinically, it is important to follow the treatment determined by the syndromes.

1. Therapeutic Effect of Acupuncture and Moxibustion

Traditional Chinese medicine holds that all matter and phenomena in the universe contain aspects of yin and yang, which are interrelated and opposed but the same entity. The theory of yin and yang is also used to explain the physiology and pathology of the human body. Under normal conditions the human body has a relative balance of yin and yang. An imbalance of yin and yang causes disease.

When a pathogenic agent invades the human body, antipathogenic agents resist it. If the antipathogenic agents are strong, the disease will be hindered. The effectiveness of acupuncture and moxibustion in treatment of disease is due mainly to regulation of yin and yang, strengthening of the body's defences and elimination of the pathogens.

Experiments of modern medicine have proved that acupuncture and moxibustion can strengthen the central nervous system, reinforcing especially the action of the sympathetic nervous system and cerebral cortex, which control all the tissues and organs of the human body. For instance, acupuncture and moxibustion can regulate the heartbeats, body temperature, blood pressure and respiration. They can relieve muscle spasms and cure numbness. They can also remove disturbance of exocrine and endocine secretions and promote secretion of the glands, such as pituitary, thyroid, parathyroid, adrenic, sweat, pancreatic and digestive.

2. Treatment Determined According to Syndromes

A disease often has a complicated cause and development, hence various symptoms and signs must be analyzed and systematized according to knowledge of the zang organs and meridians. Only in this way can one understand its nature—cold or hot, a deficiency or excess, exterior or interior, affection of meridians and internal organs. Then treatment can be determined. Our predecessors, through their practice, summarized the following rules of treatment in acu-moxibustion: The reducing method is employed for excess, the reinforcing method for deficiency, swift insertion and withdrawal of needles without retention for heat, needle retention for cold, moxibustion for deficient vital function and collapse of the yang, bloodletting for stasis.

The reducing method for excess refers to needle manipulation, i.e. strong stimulation should be used to treat some acute or paroxysmal cases in which the normal qi of the body is still of sufficient strength, the pathogenic agents are hyperactive and a severe confrontation takes place between them. Symptoms are high fever, severe pain, etc.

The reinforcing method for deficiency refers to mild stimulation by acupuncture or moxibustion applied to cases with deficiency of the normal qi. Symptoms are coughing, asthma due to weakness of the lung, palpitation, shortness of breath, etc.

Swift insertion and withdrawal of needles without retention for heat refers to inserting the needle rapidly without retention after manipulation or twirling the needle with high frequency after insertion (i.e. the reducing method). In addition, it also includes cutaneous needling or bloodletting to the Jing (Well) points on the tips of the fingers and toes. These methods are prescribed for some disorders resulting from wind heat or heat transformed from wind and cold, e.g. colds due to wind and heat, loss of consciousness due to high fever, etc.

Needles retained for cold means that the needles should be inserted for a period of time, twirling the needle intermittently or not twirling at all. In addition, moxibustion, or cupping, may also be applied to treat some diseases caused by pathogenic cold, e.g. cold due to wind and cold, rheumatic or rheumatoid arithritis resulting from excessive cold and dampness and diarrhoea due to endogenous cold.

Moxibustion for deficient qi and collapse of yang is a method for diseases resulting from a deficiency of qi, e.g. chronic dysentery, diarrhoea, prolapse of rectum. Moxibustion should be used to invigorate the body's yang. Moxibustion may also be used for profuse sweating, cold limbs and fading pulse due to a sudden collapse of yang.

Bloodletting for stasis means that disorders of stagnation and accumulation of blood resulting from traumatic injuries, erysipelas and some other factors may be treated by pricking with the filiform needle or the three-edged needle to cause bleeding, followed by cupping.

3. Selection and Combined Use of Points

Acu-moxibustion treatment is based on the function of points. Therefore, it is important to make a correct selection of them.

How to select points

(a) Selection of local and adjacent points: Each point used can treat local disorders and disorders of adjacent tissues and organs. When a certain part of the body is affected, the points located in the affected area or neighbouring areas should be prescribed for treatment. For instance, Zhongwan (CV 12) and Liangmen (S 21) are chosen to deal with gastric pain, Jiache (S 6) and Xiaguan (S 7) are punctured for toothache, Tianshu (S 25) and Qihai (CV 6) are prescribed for diarrhoea. Under normal conditions local points are taken as the main points, or local and adjacent points are combined. But if there are important organs, ulcers, or scars in the local area, the local points should not be punctured; the adjacent points should be used instead.

(b) Selection of points according to the course of the meridian: Points below the elbow or knee affect diseases occurring in the face, trunk, and tissues and organs far from them. For disorders in a meridian or its corresponding viscus the points of the involved meridian or those related to the diseased one should be prescribed for treatment.

Points pertaining to the affected meridians and organs may be selected. For instance, disorders of the lung can be treated by needling Chize (L 5), Kongzui (L 6), and Taiyuan (L 9) which are in the Lung Meridian of Hand-Taiyin. Zusanli (S 36) and Liangqiu (S 34) in the Stomach Meridian of Foot-Yangming may be used to treat disorders in the stomach. Yinmen (B 37) and Weizhong (B 40) in the Urinary Bladder Meridian of Foot-Taiyang are indicated for pain in the back and waist.

Selecting points in related channels generally means that points united externally and internally related to the diseased meridian or points that bear the same name should be selected.

Selecting points pertaining to meridians related externally and internally: For instance, Hegu (LI 4) in the Large Intestine Meridian of Hand-Yangming is chosen to treat disorders of the lung because the lung is externally and internally related to the large intestine. Shangqiu (Sp 5) and Gongsun (Sp 4) in the Spleen Meridian of Foot-Taiyin are used to treat diseases in the gastric region.

Selecting points in a meridian bearing the same name as the diseased meridian: For disorders in the liver, Neiguan (P 6) in the Pericardium Meridian of Hand-Jueyin is chosen. Taixi (K 3) and Zhaohai (K 6) in the Kidney Meridian of Foot-Shaoyin are prescribed for disorders in the heart.

Selecting points according to the course of the meridian is also known as selection of distal points. It includes choosing points on the lower part of the body, i.e. below the elbow and knee, to treat diseases on the upper part, and vice versa. For example, Houxi (SI 3) is selected to deal with pain in the neck and nape, Yongquan (K 1) is used to treat a severe case of apoplexy, and Baihui (GV 20) and Shuigou (GV 26) are selected to treat prolapse of the rectum due to chronic dysentery, back pain, respectively.

(c) Selecting points according to symptoms and signs is selection on the basis of either the doctor's experience or the patient's symptoms to treat some disorders in the nervous system or general disorders. For example, Dazhui (GV 14), Quchi (LI 11), Hegu (LI 4), Shixuan (Extra 30), and twelve Jing (Well) points are prescribed for excess syndrome with high fever. Neiguan (P 6), Daling (P 7), Yinxi (H 6), Sanyinjiao (Sp 6) and Taixi (K 3) deal with fever due to deficiency of yin. Suliao (GV 25), Shuigou (GV 26), Yongquan (K 1) and Huiyin (CV 1) are for syncope with cold limbs. Needling of Neiguan (P 6) and Zusanli (S 36) and moxibustion for Baihui (GV 20), Qihai (CV 6) and Guanyuan (CV 4) are indicated for the flaccid type of apoplexy (shock and heart failure). Yinxi (H 6), Fuliu (K 7), Hegu (LI 4) and Houxi (SI 3) are prescribed for night sweating,

Fengchi (G 31), Xinshu (B 15), Shenmen (H 7), Neiguan (P 6) and Sanyinjiao (Sp 6) for insomnia and dream-disturbed sleep. For convulsions, Hegu (LI 4), Taichong (Liv 3), and Yintang (Extra 1) are chosen. Qihai (CV 6), Dazhui (GV 14), Guanyuan (CV 4), Mingmen (GV 4), Gaohuang (B 43), and Zusanli (S 36) are used for debility, Jianshi (P 5) or Neiguan (P 6), Hegu (LI 4) and Shixuan (Extra 24) for malaria, and Geshu (B 17), Quchi (CV 6), Hegu (LI 4), Xuehai (Sp 10) and Sanyinjiao (Sp 6) for itching skin. Zhongwan (CV 12) and Fenglong (S 40) are effective for profuse sputum, Shuifen (CV 9) and Yinlingquan (Sp 9) for edema. Sifeng (Extra 29) and Zusanli (S 36) deal with infantile indigestion, and anemia can be treated by puncturing Geshu (B 17), Pishu (B 20), and Xuanzhong (B 39).

Combining points

(a) Points on the upper and lower extremities can be used simultaneously to treat disorders in the same part of the body. For instance, Neiguan (P 6) of the upper extremity is combined with Gongsun (Sp 4) of the lower limb for disorders in the heart, chest and gastric region; Hegu (LI 4) and Neiting (S 44) or Taichong (SI 11) are used in combination to deal with disorders in the head and face.

(b) Combining anterior and posterior points: Anterior refers to the chest and abdomen, while posterior means the back. Points on both parts of the body can be used jointly to treat diseases of the internal organs. For instance, disorders of the heart can be treated by puncturing Shanzhong (CV 17) on the chest and Xinshu (B 15) or Jueyinshu (B 14) on the back; Tianshu (S 25) on the abdomen and Dachangshu (B 25) on the waist are used in combination to deal with disorders of the large intestine.

(c) Combining points on the left and right: Some meridians can cross from right to left or from left to right. Therefore, disorders on the left side can be treated by puncturing points on the right and vice versa. For instance, Migraine on the right can be treated by needling Yanglingquan (G 34), Xiaxi (G 43) on the left side, and vice versa. Facial paralysis on the left is cured by selecting Hegu (LI 4) on the right.

(d) Combining points according to the external-internal relationship of the channels means points pertaining to the exterior and yang and those belonging to the interior and yin can be used simultaneously. For instance, Zusanli (S 36) and Liangqiu (S 34) in the Stomach Meridian of Foot-Yangming combined with Shangqiu (Sp 5) or Gongsun (Sp 4) in the Spleen Meridian of Foot-Taiyin are indicated for discorders of the stomach. Chize (L 5) and Taiyuan (L 9) in the lung meridian and Hegu (LI 4) in the Large Intestine Meridian are used to treat lung diseases.

(e) Combining local and distal points is used extensively in clinical practice. For most disorders of the head, face, trunk and internal organs local or adjacent points of the diseased site and distal points of the four extremities, especially those below the elbow and knee, may be prescribed in combination on the basis of the channel course. For example, the local points Zhongwan (CV 12) and Liangmen (S 21) or the adjacent point Weishu (B 21) combined with the distal points Zusanli (S 36), Neiguan (P 6) or Gongsun (Sp 4) are used to treat gastric pain.

The following list indicates combinations of local and distal points.

Table 1. Examples of Prescriptions of Local and Distal Points

Diseased area	Local and adjacent points	Distal Points Upper extremity	Distal Points Lower extremity	Other
Vertex	Baihui (GV 20) Fengchi (B 20)	Hegu (LI 4)	Taichong (Liv 3) Yongquan (K 1)	
Forehead	Yintang (Extra 1) Shangxing (GV 23) Touwei (S 8)	Hegu (LI 4)	Neiting (S 44) Jiexi (S 41)	
Temple	Shuaigu (G 8) Taiyang (Extra 2) Fengchi (G 20)	Waiguan (TE 5)	Foot Linqi (G 41) Xiaxi (G 43)	
Nape	Fengchi (G 20) Tianzhu (B 20) Dazhui (GV 4)	Houxi (SI 3)	Shenmai (B 62) Kunlun (B 60)	
Eye	Jingming (B 1) Chengqi (S 1) Muchuang (G 16) Fengchi (G 20)	Hegu (LI 4) Yanglao (SI 6)	Xingjian (Liv 2)	
Nose	Yingxiang (LI 20) Shangxing (GC 23)	Hegu (LI 4)	Neiting (S 44)	
Mouth and teeth	Dicang (S 4) Jiache (S 6) Xiguan (S 7)	Hegu (LI 4) Yangxi (LI 5)	Taichong (Liv 3) Neiting (S 44) Zhaohai (K 6)	
Tongue	Liangquan (CV 23) Yamen (GC 15)	Tongli (H 5)	Taichong (Liv 3) Taibai (Sp 3)	
Ear	Tinggong (SI 19) Ermen (TE 21) Yifeng (TE 17)	Hand Zhongzhu (TE 3) Waiguan (TE 5)	Xiaxi (G 43)	
Throat	Liangquan (CV 20) Yifeng (TE 17) Tiantu (CV 22)	Shaoshang (L 11) Hegu (LI 4)	Zhaohai (K 6)	
Lung	Feishu (B 13) Shanzhong (CV 17) Tiantu (CV 22)	Chize (Lu 5) Lieque (Lu 7) Taiyuan (Lu 9)	Taixi (K 3) Fenglong (S 40)	
Heart	Xinshu (B 15) Jueyinshu (B 14) Shanzhong (CV 17)	Neiguan (P 6) Shenmen (H 7) Jianshi (P 5) Ximen (P 4)	Gongsun (Sp 4) Sanyinjiao (Sp 6)	
Liver	Ganshu (B 19) Qimen (Liv 14)	Hand Wangu (SI 4) Zhigou (SJ 6)	Taichong (Liv 3) Yanglingquan (G 34)	
Gallbladder	Danshu (B 19) Riyue (G 24)	Zhigou (SJ 6)	Qiuxu (G 40) Yanglingquan (G 34) Taichong (Liv 3) Gallbladder	

			(Extra 35)	
Stomach	Zhongwan (CV 12) Weishu (B 21) Liangmen (S 21)	Neiguan (P 6) Hegu (LI 4)	Zusanli (S 36) Fenglong (S 40) Liangqiu (S 34) Gongsun (Sp 4)	
Intestine	Dachangshu (B 25) Xiaochangshu (B 27) Tianshu (S 25) Guanyuan (CV 4)	Hegu (LI 4) Shousanli (LI 10)	Zusanli (S 36) Shangjuxu (S 37) Xiajuxu (S 39) Lanwei (Extra 33)	
Kidney	Shenshu (B 23) Zhishi (B 52) Sanjiaoshu (B 22) Shuifen (CV 9) Qihai (CV 6)		Taixi (K 3) Fuliu (K 7) Weiyang (B 39) Sanyinjiao (Sp 6)	
Urinary bladder	Ciliao (B 32) Zhongji (CV 3)		Sanyinjiao (Sp 6) Yanglingquan (G 34)	
External genitalia	Guanyuan (CV 4) Qihai (CV 6) Zhongji (CV 3) Guilai (S 29) Ciliao (B 32) Shenshu (B 23)		Sanyinjiao (Sp 6) Ququan (Liv 8) Taichong (Liv 3) Taixi (K 3) Ligou (Liv 5) Xuehai (Sp 10)	
Anus	Changqiang (GV 1)	Kongzui (L 6)	Chengshan (B 57)	Baihui (GV 20)
Back and waist	Local points		Weizhong (B 40) Yinmen (B 37) Chengshan (B 57) Kunlun (B 60)	Renzhong (GV 20)
Chest	Local points	Neiguan (P 6) Daling (P 7) Taiyuan (L 9)	Fenglong (S 40) Taibai (Sp 3)	
Upper extremities		Jianyu (LI 15) Quchi (LI 11) Hegu (LI 4)		Jiaji points (on both sides of the spinal column at the lateral borders of each spinous process) from the fifth vertebra to the first thoracic vertebra
Lower extremities			Huantiao (G 30) Yangling (G 34) Xuanzhong (G 39)	Jiaji points from the first lumbar vertebra to the fourth sacral vertebra Fengfu (GV 16)

It is usually advisable to choose two to five points for each treatment in the methods mentioned above.

4. Specific Points and Their Applications

Some key points in the fourteen channels have their own particular properties. They can be further classified into specialized groups under certain names. Some of them are often used in clinical practice.

The Five Shu Points

In each of the twelve symmetrical channels there are five specific points located below the elbow and knee, namely Jing (Well), Xing (Spring), Shu (Stream), Jing (River) and He (Sea). Jing means the vital energy of the channel is like the water in a well. Xing means the vital energy is slightly stronger, similar to a spring. Shu means the vital energy is even stronger, flowing like a stream. Jing (River) means the vital energy is flowing like a river. He means the full strength of the vital energy, like a river flowing into the sea.

Table of the Five Shu Points

The uses of the five Shu points: Jing (Well) points are for diseases related to mental disorder and stuffiness of the epigastric region. Xing (Spring) points are for febrile diseases. Shu (Stream) points are for diseases related to the heaviness of the body and arthralgia. Jing (River) points are for cough, asthma and sore throat. He (Sea) points are for pathological changes of the intestines and stomach.

The Five Shu Points of the Yin Meridians

	Meridian	I (Wood) Jing (Well)	II (Fire) Xing (Spring)	III (Earth) Shu (Stream)	IV (Metal) Jing (River)	V (Water) He (Sea)
The three yin meridians of the hand	Lung Hand-Taiyin	Shaoshang (L 11)	Yuji (L 10)	Taiyuan (L 9)	Jingqu (L 8)	Chize (L 5)
	Pericardium Hand-Jueyin	Zhongchong (P 9)	Laogong (P 8)	Daling (P 7)	Jianshi (P 5)	Quze (P 3)
	Heart Hand-Shaoyin	Shaochong (H 9)	Shaofu (H 8)	Shenmen (H 7)	Lingdao (H 4)	Shaohai (H 3)
The three yin meridians of the foot	Spleen Foot-Taiyin	Yinbai (Sp 1)	Dadu (Sp 2)	Taibai (Sp 3)	Shangqiu (Sp 5)	Yinlingquan (Sp 9)
	Liver Foot-Jueyin	Dadun (Liv 1)	Xingjian (Liv 2)	Taichong (Liv 3)	Zhongfeng (Liv 4)	Ququan (Liv 8)
	Kidney Foot-Shaoyin	Yongquan (K 1)	Rangu (K 2)	Taixi (K 3)	Fuliu (K 7)	Yingu (K 10)

The Five Shu Points of the Yang Meridians

	Meridian	I (Metal) Jing (Well)	II (Water) Xing (Spring)	III (Wood) Shu (Stream)	IV (Fire) Jing (River)	V (Earth) He (Sea)
The three yang meridians of the hand	Large Intestine of the Hand-Yangming	Shangyang (LI 1)	Erjian (LI 2)	Sanjian (LI 3)	Yangxi (LI 5)	Quchi (LI 11)
	Sanjiao of the Hand-Shaoyang	Guanchong (TE 1)	Yemen (TE 2)	Hand-Zhongzhu (TE 3)	Zhigou (TE 6)	Tianjing (TE 10)
	Small Intestine of the Hand-Taiyang	Shaoze (SI 1)	Qiangu (SI 2)	Houxi (SI 3)	Yanggu (SI 5)	Xiaohai (SI 8)
The three yang meridians of the foot	Stomach of the Foot-Yangming	Lidui (S 45)	Neiting (S 44)	Xiangu (S 43)	Jiexi (S 41)	Zusanli (S 36)
	Gallbladder of the Foot-Shaoyang	Foot-Qiaoyin (G 44)	Xiaxi (G 43)	Foot Linqi (G 41)	Yangfu (G 38)	Yang-lingquan (G 34)
	Urinary Bladder of the Foot-Taiyang	Zhiyin (B 67)	Foot Tonggu (B 66)	Shugu (B 65)	Kunlun (B 60)	Weizhong (B 40)

Back-Shu and Front-Mu Points

Each of the zang-fu organs has a Back-Shu and Front-Mu point. These points belong to different regular or extraordinary meridians. The Back-Shu points are located in the Urinary Bladder Meridian of Foot-Taiyang along the spinal column, arranged according to the sites of the internal organs. The qi of the internal organs, meridians, and their collaterals are transported and infused to the back of the body, which pertains to yang.

The Front-Mu points are located in the chest and abdomen close to their corresponding internal organs. The qi of the internal organs, meridians and their collaterals converge in the chest and abdomen, which pertain to yin.

Table of the Back-Shu and Front-Mu Points

The Back-Shu and Front-Mu points can be used separately or in combination. Clinically, the Back-Shu points are often used in treating diseases of the five zang organs, and the Front-Mu Points are commonly used for diseases of the six fu organs. The Back-Shu points are used not only for diseases of corresponding organs, but also for diseases in associated areas. For example, the liver has its opening in the eyes, so Ganshu (B 18) can be used for diseases of the eye. The kidneys have their opening in the ears, so Shenshu (B 23) can be selected to treat ear troubles.

The Back-Shu Points and the Front-Mu Points

Back-Shu Point	Internal Organ	Front-Mu Point	Pertaining Meridian
Feishu (B 13)	Lung	Zhongfu (L 1)	Hand-Taiyin
Jueyinshu (B 14)	Pericardium	Shanzhong (CV 17)	Conception Vessel Meridian
Xinshu (B 14)	Heart	Jujue (CV 14)	Conception Vessel Meridian
Ganshu (B 18)	Liver	Qimen (Liv 14)	Foot-Jueyin
Pishu (B 20)	Spleen	Zhangmen (Liv 13)	Foot-Jueyin
Shenshu (B 23)	Kidney	Jingmen (G 25)	Foot-Shaoyang
Dachangshu (B 25)	Large Intestine	Tianshu (S 25)	Foot-Yangming
Sanjiaoshu (B 22)	Sanjiao	Shimen (CV 5)	Conception Vessel Meridian
Xiaochangshu (B 27)	Small Intestine	Guanyuan (CV 4)	Conception Vessel Meridian
Weishu (B 21)	Stomach	Zhongwan (CV 12)	Conception Vessel Meridian
Danshu (B 19)	Gallbladder	Riyue (G 24)	Foot-Shaoyang
Pangguangshu (B 28)	Urinary Bladder	Zhongji (CV 3)	Conception Vessel Meridian

Yuan (Source) and Luo (Connecting) Points

The Yuan points are places the qi of the zang-fu organs, meridians and their collaterals passes through and infuses. The Yuan points on all the yin meridians coincide with the Shu (Stream) points or the five Shu points, but each of the yang meridians has a Yuan point of its own, which always follows the Shu (Stream) Point in order. The Yuan points are close together in the wrist and ankle region. They are of great significance in diagnosis and in treatment of diseases in the meridians and zang-fu organs.

Luo points are located in the fifteen collaterals, branches of the fourteen meridians. Each of the fourteen meridians has a Luo (Connecting) point, and there are two Luo points on the spleen meridian. One is Gongsun (Sp 4) and the other is Dabao (Sp 21). Thus there are fifteen Luo points in all. Because the collaterals connect a definite pair of meridians, known as externally-internally related to one another, their points are used to treat diseases of meridians and the zang-fu organs. Clinically, the Yuan and Luo points can be used separately or in combination, but we should take the Yuan points, located in their original meridians, as the main points, with the Luo points as the secondary. For instance, if the disease is in the heart meridian, take the Yuan point—Shenmen (H 7) as the main point and the Luo point—Zhizheng (SI 7) of the small intestine meridian as the secondary point. See the table below:

Yuan (Source) and Luo (Connecting) Points

Meridian	Yuan points	Luo points
Lung Meridian of Hand-Taiyin	Taiyuan (L 9)	Lieque (L 7)
Pericardium Meridian of Hand-Jueyin	Daling (P 7)	Neiguan (P 6)
Heart Meridian of Hand-Shaoyin	Shenmen (H 7)	Tongli (H 5)
Spleen Meridian of Foot-Taiyin	Taibai (Sp 3)	Gongsun (Sp 4)
Liver Meridian of Foot-Jueyin	Taichong (Liv 3)	Ligou (Liv 5)
Kidney Meridian of Foot-Shaoyin	Taixi (K 3)	Dazhong (K 4)
Large Intestine Meridian of Hand-Yangming	Hegu (LI 4)	Pianli (LI 6)
Triple Energizer Meridian of Hand-Shaoyang	Yangchi (TE 4)	Waiguan (TE 5)
Small Intestine Meridian of Hand-Taiyang	Wangu (SI 4)	Zhizheng (SI 7)
Stomach Meridian of Foot-Yangming	Chongyang (S 42)	Fenglong (S 40)
Gallbladder Meridian of Foot-Shaoyang	Qiuxu (G 40)	Guangming (G 37)
Urinary-Bladder Meridian of Foot-Taiyang	Jinggu (B 64)	Feiyang (B 58)

The Eight Influential Points

The eight influential points are those very closely related to the zang-fu organs, qi, blood, muscles and tendons, blood vessels, bones and marrow. Any pathological changes of those tissues and organs can be treated by the relative influential point. For example, Tanzhong (CV 17), one of the eight influential points known as a qi influential point, can be used to remove the dysfunction of qi, i.e. stuffiness of the chest, shortness of breath, etc. Geshu (B 17) is an influential point of blood, which can be used in treating blood deficiency and driving away pathogenic heat from the blood. The influential point Zhangmen (Liv 13) is used to treat diseases of the zang organs.

The Eight Influential Points

Tissue	Influential point
Associated with zang organs	Zhangmen (Liv 13)
Associated with fu organs	Zhongwan (CV 12)
Associated with qi	Shanzhong (CV 17)
Associated with blood	Geshu (B 17)
Associated with sinew	Yanglingquan (G 34)
Associated with vessels	Taiyuan (L 9)

Associated with bone	Dashu (B 11)
Associated with marrow	Xuanzhong (G 39)

The Eight Confluent Points

In the twelve regular meridians there are eight points in the extremities that are connected to the eight extraordinary meridians. These points are often divided into four groups. Each has its own therapeutic properties. For instance, Neiguan (P 6) and Gongsun (Sp 4) join as one group for illness of chest, heart and stomach. Lieque (L 7) used with Zhaohai (K 6) as a group can treat diseases of the lung, throat, chest and diaphragm.

The Eight Confluent Points and Their Uses

Confluent points	Pertaining to regular meridian	Communicating with extraordinary meridian	Use (Portion of the body)
Gongsun (Sp 4)	Spleen	Chong	Heart, chest,
Neiguan (P 6)	Pericardium	Yinwei	stomach
Houxi (SI 3)	Small intestine	Governor Vessel	Neck, shoulder, back,
Shenmai (B 62)	Urinary bladder	Yangqiao	inner canthus, ear region
Foot Linqi (G 41)	Gallbladder	Dai	Outer canthus, cheek, shoulder,
Waiguan (TE 5)	Sanjiao	Yangwei	neck, mastoid region
Lieque (L 7)	Lung	Conception Vessel	Lung, throat,
Zhaohai (K 6)	Kidney	Yinqiao	chest, diaphragm

The Xi (Cleft) Points

The Xi (Cleft) point is the spot where the qi of the meridians converges deeply between the bones and muscles. Clinically, these points are more often used in acute diseases. For instance, Kongzui (L 6), one of the Xi points in Lung Meridian, can be used in treating hemoptysis; Ximen (P 4), the Xi point in the Pericardium Meridian, is used for cardiac pain and stuffiness of the chest; gastric pain can be treated by the Xi point —Liangqiu (S 34) in Stomach Meridian. Each of the twelve regular meridians has a Xi point, and the Yinwei, Yangwei, Yinjiao and Yangjiao extraordinary meridians have one too, making sixteen in all.

The Xi (Cleft) Points

Meridian	Xi Point
Lung Meridian of Hand-Taiyin	Kongzui (L 6)
Pericardium Meridian of Hand-Jueyin	Ximen (P 4)
Heart Meridian of Hand-Shaoyin	Yinxi (H 6)
Large Intestine Meridian of Hand-Yangming	Wenliu (LI 7)
Small-Intestine Meridian of Hand-Taiyang	Yanglao (SI 6)
Triple Energizer Meridian of Hand-Shaoyang	Huizong (TE 7)
Spleen Meridian of Foot-Taiyin	Diji (Sp 8)
Liver Meridian of Foot-Jueyin	Foot-Zhongdu (Liv 6)
Kidney Meridian of Foot-Shaoyin	Shuiquan (K 5)
Stomach Meridian of Foot-Yangming	Liangqiu (S 34)
Gallbladder Meridian of Foot-Shaoyang	Waiqiu (G 36)
Urinary-Bladder Meridian of Foot-Taiyang	Jinmen (B 63)
Yinwei Meridian	Zhubin (K 9)
Yangwei Meridian	Yangjiao (G 35)
Yinqiao Meridian	Jiaoxin (K 8)
Yangqiao Meridian	Fuyang (B 59)

The Lower He (Sea) Points

The six lower He (Sea) points are located in the lower extremities where the qi of the meridians communicates with its fu organ. These points are mostly used in treating diseases in the fu organs. For instance, diseases in the large intestine can be treated by the lower He point—Shangjuxu (S 37). The lower He point—Xiajuxu (St 39) can be used in treating diseases in the small intestine.

The Lower He (Sea) Points of the Six Fu Organs

Six fu organs	Lower He point	Yang meridian of foot
Stomach	Zusanli (S 36)	Foot-Yangming
Large intestine	Shangjuxu (S 37)	
Small intestine	Xiajuxu (S 39)	
Triple energizer	Weiyang (B 39)	Foot-Taiyang
Urinary bladder	Weizhong (B 40)	
Gallbladder	Yanglingquan (G 34)	Foot-Shaoyang

Chapter II
Treatment of Common Diseases with Acupuncture and Moxibustion

1. Apoplexy, or Stroke

Apoplexy is characterized mainly by sudden coma, sometimes accompanied by distortion of eyes and mouth, hemiplegia, speech defect, and so on. It is usually due to hyperactivity of the liver yang and upward flow of qi and blood, resulting in dizziness, numbness of the fingertips and such prodromal signs of an attack. Simulating wind in its rapid change and abruptness, it is called in Chinese "stricken by wind," because the onset is abrupt, the condition critical and the disease tends to worsen quickly.

Known as cerebrovascular accident in Western medicine, it includes cerebral hemorrhage, thrombosis and embolism.

Etiology and Pathology

Medical practitioners differ over the cause of the disease, but most hold that it is often induced by excessive anxiety and anger, alcohol addiction, overtiredness, excessive sexual activities and so on, against a background of breakdown of the equilibrium of yin and yang, leading to an agitation of wind and sudden preponderance of heart fire. The wind and fire combine, forcing qi and blood to rush upwards and the phlegm to block meridians. Dysfunction of the zang-fu organs, meridians and collaterals occur. Disturbance of the yin and yang brings about blockage or tense syndrome, while separation causes collapse or flaccid syndrome or obstruction of meridians, impeding normal circulation of qi. Clinically, depending on the severity of the disease, there are two types of stroke, meridian stroke and zang-fu stroke, which is the point of departure in differentiation and treatment.

Differentiation

A. Meridian Stroke

The meridians and collaterals are affected without the zang-fu organs being involved, or the function of the zang-fu organs has recovered, yet there is still obstruction in the meridians and collaterals. Manifestations are hemiplegia, numbness, rigid tongue and speech defect or distortion of the mouth and eyes, floating, taut and slippery pulse.

B. Zang-fu Stroke

The affected area is in the zang-fu organs. Manifestations are sudden coma, hemiplegia, speech defect, distortion of mouth and eyes, and so on. Zang-fu stroke can also be divided into blockage or tense syndrome and collapse or flaccid syndrome in accordance with different causes.

(1) Blockage Syndrome

It is usually due to upward rush of qi and fire, blood stagnation in the upper portion of the body, agitation of wind in the liver, and excessive phlegm. Coma, lockjaw, clenched fists, flushed face, hoarse breathing, rattling in the throat, retention of urine and feces, taut, slippery and rapid pulse may occur.

(2) Collapse

It is caused by feebleness of primordial qi and a sudden breakdown of the kidneys' vital function, known as original yang, manifestations of which are eyes closed and mouth agape, hands relaxed, incontinence of urine, diminished breathing, cold limbs, and feeble pulse. There may be excessive sweating, blushing, fading pulse, indicating the running down of the original yang—a sign of imminent death.

Treatment

A. Body Acupuncture

(1) Meridian Stroke

(a) Hemiplegia

Method: Main points are in Foot-Yangming meridians, subsidiary points in Taiyang and Shaoyang meridians. Generally, needling is applied to the healthy side, or the healthy side first and then the affected side, known as "reinforcing the healthy side and reducing the affected side."

Prescription:

Upper extremity: Jianyu (LI 15), Quchi (LI 11), Waiguan (TE 5), Hegu (LI 4).

Lower extremity: Huantiao (G 30), Yanglingquan (G 34), Zusanli (S 36), Jiexi (S 41), Kunlun (B 60).

Explanation: Treatment is centred on the Yangming meridian, in which ample qi and blood circulate. Points of the Hand- and Foot-Yangming meridians are selected to adjust the function of the meridians and promote smooth circulation of qi and blood.

(b) Facial Paralysis

Method: Main points are Hand- and Foot-Yangming and Foot-Jueyin meridians. In the early stage of the disease needling is applied only to the affected side, but to both sides in a long-standing case.

Prescription: Dicang (S 4), Jiache (S 6), Hegu (LI 4), Neiting (P 6), Taichong (Liv 3).

Explanation: The Hand- and Foot-Yangming and Foot-Jueyin meridians all go upward to the face and head. The local meridian qi is regulated by needling the adjacent points—Dicang (S 4), Jiache (S 6). The whole meridian qi is regulated by needling the distal points—Hegu (LI 4), Neiting (P 6) and Taichong (Liv 3).

Modification: Renzhong (GV 26), Yangbai (G 14) and Xiaguan (S 7) on the affected side are added.

(2) Zang-Fu Stroke

(a) Blockage Syndrome

Method: Main points are in the Governor Vessel Meridian and the Jing (Well) points. Use filiform needle or prompt pricking bleeding.

Prescription: Renzhong (GV 26), twelve Jing (Well) points, Taichong (Liv 3),

Fenglong (S 40), Laogong (P 8).

Explanation: To check the liver, expel the pathogenic wind, repel fire and eliminate "phlegm" for resuscitation. The onset of the disease is due to a sudden agitation of the liver yang, upward rush of qi and blood, and at the same time the Heart Meridian is obstructed by "phlegm"—a pathogenic agent. The treatment is aimed at resuscitation and removal of excessive heat by needling the twelve Jing (Well) points until there is bleeding and Renzhong (GV 26) with the reducing method. Since the Liver Meridian runs up to the vertex on the head, it is essential to needle Taichong (Liv 3) to relieve the abnormal flow of the liver qi and bring down the hyperfunction of the liver. The spleen is the source of formation of "phlegm," retention of which causes the dysfunction of the spleen in its transportation and transformation. Fenglong (S 40), located at the branch collateral of the Foot-Yangming Meridian, is used to activate the smooth circulation of qi in the meridians of the spleen and stomach and eliminate "phlegm." Xing (Spring) points are indicated in febrile disease; Laogong (P 8), located in the Pericardium Meridian of Hand-Jueyin, is used to drive pathogenic heat from the Pericardium Meridian.

Modifications:

Clenched jaws: Jiache (S 6) and Hegu (LI 4) are added.

Speech defect: Yamen (GV 15), Lianquan (CV 23), Tongli (H 5) and Guanchong (TE 1) are added.

(b) Collapse

Method: Conception Vessel Meridian points are main points, with moxibustion.

Prescription: Guanyuan (CV 4), Shenjue (CV 8) (indirect moxibustion with salt).

Explanation: The Conception Vessel Meridian is the sea of the yin meridians; Guanyuan (CV 4), the intersecting point of the Conceptional Vessel Meridian and the three yin meridians, is the site through which the vital energy flows out. It is a point communicating with the fire of the Life Gate and thought to be a yang point within yin. Rescuing yang by selecting points pertaining to yin is necessary to recapture yang. Shenjue (CV 8), located at the umbilicus, in the Conception Vessel Meridian, is connected with the primordial qi. Moxibustion applied with a big moxa cone to these two points is desirable for restoration of the diminished yang.

B. Scalp Acupuncture

Main points are in the motor region of the opposite side, combined with points on the motor-sensory region of the foot. The speech region can be used for speech defect. The patient should be treated as early as possible. Generally, a marked result is seen in cerebral thrombosis.

C. Electroacupuncture

Two to three pairs of the above-mentioned points on the extremities are selected. A lifting and thrusting movement should be applied after the needles are inserted, allowing the needling sensation to spread to the distal end. Then an electroacupuncture apparatus is connected to the needle and the intensity of stimulation is increased gradually for about thirty seconds. After ceasing stimulation awhile, the apparatus works for another thirty seconds; this is repeated three or four times. The patient feels numb, and a rhythmical contraction of the related muscle groups appears.

Remarks

(1) Acupuncture and moxibustion on Fengshi (G 31) and Zusanli (S 36) should be given to obese older people who have tingling and numbness in the fingertips caused by hyperactivity of the liver yang and deficiency of qi. Special concern is given to daily life. This is considered a prophylactic way to prevent attack.

(2) Patients should be guided to do some slight exercise to recover function of the paralysed limbs; at the same time remedial massage and physiotherapy should be applied.

(3) Comprehensive treatment should be given to cerebrovascular accident at the acute stage.

2. The Common Cold

The common cold is an affection due to exogenous pathogenic factors, often experienced during all four seasons. Particularly, it occurs during the changeable weather of winter or spring. A mild case is called "injured by wind," or a common cold, while a severe one is known as a seasonal common cold.

Etiology and Pathology

The common clod usually occurs when the body's resistance is low and the weather changes suddenly. The person fails to adapt himself, and the pathogenic cold or heat invades the lungs from the exterior via the body's surface or the mouth and nose. A group of symptoms and signs in the lungs appear. Because the exogenous pathogenic factors are different and individuals have different reactions to them, clinical manifestations vary. The cold type of the common cold is due to invasion of the body's surface by cold, resulting in a closing of pores over the body's surface and impaired function of the lung qi. The heat type is due to pathogenic heat scorching of the lungs, which causes opening of the pores over the body's surface and dysfunction of the lung qi.

Differentiation

(1) Common cold due to pathogenic wind-cold: It is marked by headache, sore limbs, nasal obstruction and runny nose, cough with expectoration of dilute sputum, fever (sometimes), aversion to cold, absence of sweat, unstable, tense pulse, thin, white tongue coating.

(2) Common cold due to pathogenic wind-heat: It is manifested by fever, sweating, slight aversion to cold, cough with expectoration of mucoid sputum, sore throat, thirst, dry feeling of the nose, unstable, rapid pulse, thin, slightly yellow tongue coating.

Treatment

A. Body Acupuncture

(1) Wind-cold type

Method: Main points are in the Hand-Taiyin, Hand-Yangming and Foot-Taiyang meridians. Shallow puncture and the reducing method are used, but even reinforcing and reducing methods or moxibustion is employed for people with weak constitutions.

Prescription: Lieque (L 7), Fengmen (B 12), Fengchi (G 20), Hegu (LI 4).

Explanation: The treatment aims at elimination of the exogenous pathogenic wind-cold. Since the lungs are closely related to the skin and hair, when the cold pathogenic agent invades the surface of the body, shallow needling on Lieque (L 7) is to disseminate the lung qi and check coughing. As the Taiyang Meridian dominates the function of the superficial portion of the body, Fengmen (B 12) is needled to relieve such symptoms as fever, aversion to cold, headache and limb soreness by regulating qi flow in the Taiyang Meridian and expelling wind-cold. Fengchi (B 20), the point where the Foot-Shaoyang and Yangwei meridians meet, is selected to relieve the exterior symptoms, as the Yangwei Meridian dominates yang and the body's surface. The Taiyin Meridian is united with the Yangming Meridian in their functional yoke, in which the former represents the inner side, the latter the outer side; therefore Hegu (LI 4) is needled to eliminate pathogenic agents and relieve exterior symptoms. The four points mentioned above are used together to remove the pathogenic wind-cold and keep the lung unobstructed. If cupping therapy is applied to Feishu (B 13) and Fengmen (B 12), the pathogenic wind-cold is driven away.

(2) Wind-heat type

Method: Main points are in the Hand-Taiyin, Hand-Yangming and Hand-Shaoyang meridians, and shallow puncture with the reducing method is used.

Prescription: Dazhui (GV 14), Quchi (LI 11), Hegu (LI 4), Yuji (L 10), Waiguan (TE 5).

Explanation: The treatment aims at dispelling the pathogenic wind-heat and making the lung qi flow downward. The Governor Vessel Meridian, where Dazhui (GV 14) is located, is the "sea" of all the yang meridians, the site where the yang meridians meet. Dazhui (GV 14) is selected to expel the exogenous pathogenic agent and relieve fever. Since the Hand-Yangming Meridian is united with the Hand-Taiyin Meridian in their functional yoke, in which the former represents the outer side and the latter represents the inner side, Hegu (LI 4), the source point, and Quchi (LI 11), the sea point, of the Hand-Yangming Meridian are selected to promote the functional activities of the lungs and bring down fever. Yuji (L 10) is selected to reduce the fire in the lungs, ease the throat and check soreness. Waiguan (TE 5), the connecting point of the Hand-Shaoyang Meridian, where the Yangwei Meridian crosses, is used to dispel the exogenous pathogenic agents and bring down fever. The five points used together can eliminate the pathogenic wind-heat and help restore smooth circulation of the lung qi.

B. Ear Acupuncture

Main points: Lung, Internal Nose, Adrenal, Subcortex.

Method: Moderate stimulation is given with needle twirling for two to three minutes and needle retention for another thirty to sixty minutes. Pharynx and Tonsil are added for cases of sore throat.

Remarks

Correct diagnosis should be made because there are similarities between the symptoms of common cold and some early-stage infectious diseases.

3. Heat Stroke

Heat stroke is an acute illness occurring in summer, often caused by prolonged exposure to high temperatures or a blazing sun. In view of the varied manifestations of the disease, different terms are given, namely, "summer-heat injury" (a mild case), "heat exhaustion" and "summer-heat convulsions" (severe cases).

This disease includes thermoplegia, heat spasm and sunstroke.

Etiology and Pathology

Heat stroke is usually due to invasion of the body by summer heat and summer dampness, combined with other pathogenic agents, when one is in a debilitated state. The summer heat accumulates on the surface of the body and prevents sweating, which causes the accumulated pathogenic heat to invade the pericardium, resulting in high fever and loss of consciousness. High fever often brings about contracture of tendons and muscles, or spasm, known as "wind stirring." In case of injury of qi and essence there may be critical conditions such as profuse sweating, cold limbs, shortness of breath and fading pulse.

Differentiation

(1) Mild case: It is marked by hot sensation of the body, little sweating, dizziness, headache, distress, nausea, extreme thirst, lassitude, sleepiness, white, sticky tongue coating, soft, rapid pulse.

(2) Severe case: When summer heat invades the pericardium, manifestations are high fever, extreme thirst, dry lips, scorching sensation of the skin, irritability, loss of consciousness, contracture of tendons and muscles, spasm, reddened tongue with yellow coating, full and rapid pulse. In case of collapse of qi and essence, there may be pallor, sweating, shortness of breath, dropping of blood pressure, extremely cold limbs, loss of consciousness, convulsion, red tongue, proper with yellow coating, thin, rapid pulse.

Treatment

A. Body Acupuncture

(1) Mild case

Method: Main points are in Governor Vessel and Hand-Yangming meridians, associated with the reducing method.

Prescription: Dazhui (GV 14), Quchi (LI 11), Hegu (LI 4), Neiguan (P 6).

Explanation: Dazhui (GV 14) is a juncture of the Governar Vessel Meridian and all the yang meridians. Quchi (LI 11) and Hegu (LI 4) pertain to the Yangming Meridian. The three points are selected to clear up summer heat. Neiguan (P 6), connected with the Yinwei Meridian, which goes along the abdomen, harmonizes the stomach and lowers the stomach qi to ease the chest and eliminate nausea.

(2) Severe case

Method: Main points are in the Governor Vessel and Conception Vessel Meridians. The reducing method is used when the pericardium is invaded by summer heat. Moxibustion is given to those who suffer from collapse of qi and essence.

Prescription: Baihui (GV 20), Renzhong (GV 26), Shixuan (Extra 30), Quze (P 3), Weizhong (B 39), Yanglingquan (G 34), Chengshan (B 57), Shenque (CV 8), Guanyuan (CV 4).

Explanation: Summer heat, a pathogenic agent of yang nature, tends to attack the pericardium, causing loss of consciousness. Baihui (GV 20) and Renzhong (GV 26) are used for resuscitation by clearing the pathogenic heat. Shixuan (Extra 30), a junction of yin and yang meridians, is selected to harmonize yin and yang and promote resuscitation. Quze (P 3), the sea point of the Hand-Jueyin Meridian, and Weizhong (B 39), the sea point of the Foot-Taiyang Meridian, are pricked until bleeding to remove summer heat from the blood.

In case of contracture of tendons and muscles, Yanglingquan (B 34), the influential point of tendons and muscles, and Chengshan (B 57) are used to relax tendons and muscles and relieve spasm.

In case of collapse of qi and essence, manifested by such critical conditions as sweating, cold limbs, and faint pulse, immediate moxibustion is applied to Shenque (CV 8) and Guanyuan (CV 4) for emergency treatment. The selection of the two points in the Conception Vessel Meridian is to regain yang after reinforcing yin. Renzhong (CV 26) and Shixuan (Extra 30) are sometimes selected for promoting resuscitation.

Modification: For cases of thirst Jinjin (Extra 10) and Yuye (Extra 9) are added to clear up heat and strengthen the production of body fluids.

B. Scraping Therapy

It is advisable for mild cases of heat stroke to scrape the patient's neck, back, shoulder and arm regions, the fossa of the elbow and popliteus, etc., with a smooth porcelain spoon moistened with clean water or vegetable oil until a purplish-red colour appears.

C. Ear Acupuncture

Main points: Subcortex, Heart, Adrenal, Occiput.

Method: Strong stimulation is given with needle twirling for five minutes and retention for thirty minutes. Other points may be selected or a bleeding method on the ear apex adopted according to different symptoms and signs.

Remarks

(1) Measures for heat stroke prevention should be taken in time. (2) Remove victims of heat stroke to a place with good ventilation and give cold, moist compressions, alcohol bath, cold beverage, etc. (3) For severe cases with critical conditions of circulation, dehydration, coma, etc., emergency treatment with both Chinese and Western therapy should be given immediately. (4) Correct diagnosis should be made for epidemic encephalitis B, cerebral malaria and heat stroke for cases with coma.

4. Cough

Coughing is a principal manifestation of pulmonary affection. There are two kinds of cough: cough due to exogenous pathogenic factors and cough due to internal injury from disturbance of the zang-fu function.

Coughing often accompanies infection of the upper respiratory tract, bronchitis, bronchiectasis, pulmonary tuberculosis, etc.

Etiology and Pathology

Causative agents are exogenous or endogenous. Exogenous factors are pathogenic wind-cold, wind-heat or dry heat, which attacks the lungs through the mouth, nose and skin. The lungs are closely related to the skin and hair, and their opening is the nose. Invasion of the lungs prevents them from performing their function of dispersing. Also, the lungs may be affected by other diseased zang-fu organs. For example, dampness due to deficiency in the spleen turns into phlegm, which goes up to the lungs and impedes the descending function of them, finally coughing presents. Or when the lungs are scorched by abundant fire from stagnated lung qi, then coughing occurs owing to the dysfunction of the lungs in descending.

Differentiation

A. Exogenous Agents

Wind-heat type: Manifested by cough with expectoration of yellow sputum, heat sensation of the body, headache, dryness of the mouth, sore throat, thin, yellow tongue coating, unstable, rapid pulse.

B. Endogenous Agents

(1) Invasion of the lungs by phlegm dampness: Complaints are cough with expectoration of mucoid sputum, chest distress, poor appetite, white, sticky tongue coating, lingering smooth pulse.

(2) The lung scorched by liver fire: Symptoms are cough, chest and hypochondriac pain, coughing due to regurgitation of qi, scanty mucoid sputum, blushing, yellow tongue coating with scanty saliva, taut, rapid pulse.

Treatment

A. Acupuncture and Moxibustion

(1) Exogenous agents

Method: Main points are in Hand-Taiyin and Hand-Yangming Meridians. Shallow puncture with the reducing method is applied. Strong stimulation is given to cases of wind-heat, or retention of needles associated with moxibustion is given for cases of wind-cold.

Prescription: Feishu (B 13), Lieque (L 7), Hegu (LI 4).

Explanation: Because the lungs dominate the skin and hair and control the surface of the body, it is advisable to give shallow puncture. The Hand-Yangming Meridian is united with the Hand-Taiyin Meridian in their functional yoke, in which the former takes the outward side. Selection of Lieque (L 7), the connecting point, Hegu (LI 4), the source point, in combination with Feishu (B 13) strengthens the dispersing effect of the lungs and relieves the exterior symptoms so as to restore the function of the lungs.

Modification: For cases of swelling and soreness in the throat Shaoshang (L 11) and Chize (L 5) are added. For cases of fever and aversion to cold Dazhui (GV 14) and Waiguan (TE 5) are added.

(2) Endogenous agents

a. Invasion of the lungs by phlegm

Method: Main points are in the Hand- and Foot-Taiyin meridians. The even movement method, with or without moxibustion, is applied.

Prescription: Feishu (B 13), Taiyuan (L 9), Zhangmen (Liv 13), Taibai (Sp 3), Fenglong (S 40).

Explanation: Taiyuan (L 9), the source point of the Lung Meridian, is where the original qi corresponding to the lung is infused. Selection of Taibai (Sp 3), the source point of the Spleen Meridian, Feishu (UB 13), Zhangmen (Liv 13) and Taiyuan (L 9) strengthens the transporting function of the spleen and promotes the normal flow of the lung qi. This is known as "simultaneous treatment of the secondary and primary aspect of a disease," for the spleen is a source for producing sputum. Selection of Fenglong (S 40), the connecting point of the Foot-Yangming Meridian, is to regulate the function of the spleen and stomach. The body fluids can disperse freely, finally removing the phlegm.

b. Scorching of the lungs by liver fire

Method: Main points are in the Hand-Taiyin and Foot-Jueyin meridians. The reducing method for points in the Foot-Jueyin Meridian and the even movement method for points in the Hand-Taiyin Meridian are used.

Prescription: Feishu (B 13), Chize (L 5), Yanglingquan (B 34), Taichong (Liv 3).

Explanation: Needling applied to Feishu (B 13) regulates the function of the lungs. Chize (L 5), the sea point of the Lung Meridian, needled with the reducing method can clear up excessive heat in the lungs. Yanglingquan (B 34) and Taichong (Liv 3) remove the pathogenic heat from the liver and Gallbladder Meridians. In this way the lung yin is not scorched.

B. Ear Acupuncture

Main points: Trachea, Lung, Ear Shenmen, Occiput.

Method: Treatment is given every day or every other day. Needles are retained for thirty to sixty minutes; ten treatments constitute a course. For cases of acute bronchitis, Adrenal and Sympathetic Nerve are added. For cases of chronic bronchitis, Spleen and Kidney are added.

C. Point Injection

Main points: Dingchuan (Extra 17), Dazhu (B 11), Fengmen (B 12), Feishu (B 13).

Method: 0.5 ml vitamin B_1 solution or placental solution is injected into Feishu (B 13) for each treatment, and a pair of points, from above to below, alternately, is selected for each treatment. Treatment is given every other day; twenty times constitutes a course. It is most helpful for chronic bronchitis.

D. Point-embedding Therapy

Main points: Dazhui (GV 14), Dingchuan (Extra 17), Feishu (B 13), Xinshu (B 15), Geshu (B 17).

Modification: For shortness of breath Dingchuan (Extra 17) is added.

The aged and asthenic patient: Gaohuang (B 43), Zusanli (S 36) and others are added. Generally, point-embedding therapy is given once each month. The course is decided according to conditions.

Remarks

Cough often occurs in various kinds of respiratory-system diseases. The diagnosis must be correct and medication should be given in some cases.

5. Asthma

Asthma is a common disease marked by recurrent attacks. It manifests itself in two forms, wheezing (*xiao*,哮) and panting (*chuan*, 喘), the former a throat rattle and the latter shortness of breath, as stated in the *Commentary on Medicine*. However, the two conditions usually occur simultaneously and the causes and pathological changes are similar, so they will be described together here.

Asthma includes bronchial asthma, asthmatic bronchitis, and obstructive pulmonary emphysema.

Etiology and Pathology

Retention of phlegm and fluid in the lungs is the primary cause of the disease. Early affection is often seen in children because of repeated affection of seasonal pathogenic agents. For adults it is caused by persistent coughing. Other causes of the disease include the internal production and retention of phlegm and fluid in the lungs brought about by intake of salty, greasy food or fish, shrimp and crab by someone with lowered functioning of the spleen and stomach, or by affection of the pathogenic wind-cold associated with emotional disturbance and overstrain. The qi passage is blocked, causing the lungs to fail to work normally and producing cough, wheezing and rattling.

The acute stage is considered the "excess type" due to the stagnation of qi and accumulation of phlegm, which obstructs the qi passage. Recurrent attacks consume the vital essence of the lungs and impede the function of the spleen and kidney. That is why weakness usually occurs during remission.

Differentiation

The main manifestations are short, quick breathing and a wheezing sound in the throat. In severe cases the patient has to open his mouth and raise his shoulders in breathing. The condition falls into two categories.

(1) Excess type: Caused by exogenous wind-cold marked by cough with expectoration of dilute sputum, chills, anhidrosis, headache, thirstlessness, unstable, tense pulse, thin, white tongue coating. If it is caused by phlegm and heat, the manifestations are choking cough with expectoration of mucoid and thick yellow sputum, chest distress and pain or coughing, fever, thirst, constipation, smooth, rapid pulse, thick yellow tongue coating.

(2) Deficiency type: Caused by deficiency of lung qi due to prolonged illness, marked by short, quick breathing, weak, low voice, sweating on exertion, pale tongue, thin, rapid or weak pulse. In protracted cases, such that the kidney is too weak to receive qi, it is manifested by shortness of breath on exertion, low spirits, hidrosis, cold limbs, deep, soft pulse.

Treatment

A. Body Acupuncture

(1) Excess type:

Method: Main points are in the Hand-Taiyin Meridian. The reducing method is applied, with moxibustion for cases of wind-cold. Points in the Foot-Yangming Meridian are selected for cases due to phlegm and heat, without moxibustion.

Prescription: Shanzhong (CV 17), Lieque (L 7), Feishu (B 13), Chize (L 5).

Wind cold: Fengmen (B 12); phlegm and heat: Fenglong (S 40); severe cases: Tiantu (V 22), Dingchuan (Extra 17).

Explanation: Lieque (L 7) and Chize (L 5) strengthen the smooth flow of qi in the Hand-Taiyin Meridian. Fengmen (B 12) and Feishu (B 13), pertaining to the Foot-Taiyang Meridian, are located near the lung and taken to ease the troubled lung and dispel wind. Shanzhong (CV 17) is the influential point of qi, and Fenglong (S 40) is on a collateral of the stomach. The two points are used with the reducing method to sooth qi flow and resolve sputum and heat in nature. Tiantu (CV 22) and Dingchuan (Extra 17), local points, are taken to reduce lung qi and relieve panting.

(2) Deficiency type:

Method: Strengthen the lung and kidney qi with the reinforcing method, or apply moxibustion if necessary.

Prescription: Feishu (B 13), Gaohuang (B 43), Qihai (CV 6), Shenshu (B 23), Zusanli (S 36), Taiyuan (L 9), Taixi (K 3).

Explanation: Taiyuan (L 9) and Taixi (K 3), the source points of the lung and kidney meridians, replenish the qi of the lungs and kidneys. Moxibustion applied to Feishu (B 13) and Gaohuang (B 43) promotes lung qi, while needling on Shenshu (B 23) and Qihai (CV 6) fills up the kidney qi. Abundant qi of the lung and kidney strengthens the descending and ascending function. Zusanli (S 36) regulates the stomach qi, which is the source of transforming food into useful substances. Thus the essence of food is transferred to the lungs, giving the lung qi the ability to defend itself.

B. Ear Acupuncture

Main points: Pingchuan, Adrenal, Lung, Shenmen, Subcortex, Endocrine, Sympathetic Nerve, Occiput (several points may be applied at the onset to alleviate asthma).

C. Cutaneous Needling

Method: Cutaneous needling applied to the thenar eminence and the forearm region where the Hand-Taiyin Meridian goes or to both sternocleidomastoids for fifteen minutes may relieve asthma.

D. Point Injection

Method: 0.5 to 1 ml placental solution is injected into two Huatuo Jiaji points located between the first and sixth thoracic vertebra for each treatment. The points are above or below, alternately, every day, and the therapy is often used during remission.

E. Moxibustion

Main points: Dazhui (GV 14), Fengmen (B 12), Feishu (B 13), Shanzhong (CV 17).

Method: Indirect wheat-grain moxibustion is applied to the points. Three to five cones are burned each time at each point at ten-day intervals. Three treatments constitute a course. It is usually given on hot summer days and is most helpful during remission.

F. Point-embedding Therapy

See also under "Cough"

Remarks

(1) For cases of asthma complicated by bronchitis the bronchitis should be treated

after the asthma is relieved. (2) Medication should be given to severe or persistent cases. (3) Prevention should come first. When the weather is getting cold, patients should wear warm clothes; if allergic to certain substances, they should keep away from them.

6. Vomiting and Hiccups

Vomiting is a common clinical manifestation in a number of disorders. The stomach qi goes upward, resulting from pathogenic wind-cold, summer heat, dampness, damp and phlegm, dyspepsia and perversive flow of the liver qi.

Vomiting often accompanies such diseases as acute gastritis, hepatitis, pyloric spasm or obstruction, cardiospasm, pancreatitis, and cholecystitis.

Etiology and Pathology

Normal function of the stomach is to send the food essence upward and the waste downward with the help of the spleen. If the stomach is attacked by pathogenic agents, it fails to propel the food downwards. Vomiting results from the adverse flow of the stomach qi, retention of dampness and phlegm in the spleen and stomach, the eating of too much raw, cold or greasy food, leading to failure of the middle burner to carry out its function, deficiency of qi in the middle burner, impeding its normal digestion, caused by hypofunction of transportation and transformation, emotional depression, or invasion of the stomach by an abnormal flow of the liver qi, giving rise to an upward rush of the stomach qi.

Differentiation

Invasion of the epigastric region by pathogenic cold is manifested by vomiting of watery substance, vomiting immediately after eating, white tongue coating, slow pulse, preference for warmth and aversion to cold, and loose stool. Retention of pathogenic heat in the body is often marked by vomiting after a full meal, acid fermented vomitus, thirst, preference for cold and aversion to heat, constipation, yellow tongue coating, and rapid pulse. Retention of dampness and phlegm is often manifested by stuffiness in the chest, dizziness, vomiting of dilute phlegm, palpitation, white tongue coating, smooth pulse. Retention of undigested food is marked by epigastric and abdominal distention or pain, aggravated by intake of food, foul belching, constipation, foul gas, thick, sticky tongue coating, and forceful pulse. Invasion of the stomach by the liver qi is often manifested by hypochondriac pain, acid regurgitation, tense pulse. Weakness of the stomach is manifested by intermittent vomiting, poor appetite, slight, loose stools, general lassitude, weak pulse, thin, mucoid tongue coating.

Treatment

A. Body Acupuncture

Method: Main points are in the Foot-Yangming Meridian. For cases of excessive cold retain the needle, combined with moxibustion. For cases of excessive heat give quick needling without moxibustion. For cases of invasion of the stomach by the liver qi, needle points in the Foot-Jueyin Meridian with the reducing method and points in the Foot-Yangming Meridian with the reinforcing method. For cases of deficiency in the middle burner, it is advisable to needle with the reinforcing method and strengthen the spleen qi.

Prescription: Zhongwan (CV 12), Neiguan (P 6), Zusanli (S 36), Gongsun (Sp 4).

Secondary points for:

Vomiting due to heat: Hegu (LI 4), Jinjin (Extra 10), Yuye (Extra 9).

Vomiting due to cold: Shangwan (CV 13), Weishu (B 21).

Vomiting due to damp and phlegm: Shanzhong (CV 17), Fenglong (S 40).

Vomiting due to retardation of food: Xiawan (CV 10), Xuanji (CV 21).

Vomiting due to invasion of the stomach by the liver qi: Yanglingquan (G 34), Taichong (Liv 3).

Vomiting due to deficiency in the middle burner: Pishu (B 20), Zhangmen (Liv 13).

Explanation: Zhongwan (CV 12), the Front-Mu point of the stomach, Weishu (B 21), the Back-Shu point of the Gallbladder Meridian, Zusanli (S 36), the sea point of the Stomach Meridian are taken together to make the stomach qi go downward. Neiguan (P 6) is the connecting point of the Hand-Jueyin Meridian, descending through the diaphragm to the abdomen and connecting successively the triple burners and the confluent point of the Yinwei Meridian. The Yinwei Meridian dominates the interior of the whole body, therefore selection of Neiguan (P 6) promotes the smooth flow of the qi in the upper and middle burners. Gongsun (Sp 4) belongs to the Spleen Meridian of Foot-Taiyin and is also the confluent point of the Chong Meridian. The spleen is united with the stomach in their functional yoke, in which it takes the inner side. Gongsun (Sp 4) regulates the middle burner and pacifies the rebel qi. Moxibustion to Shangwan (CV 13), which is located on the upper portion of the stomach, warms the stomach and removes cold. Needling Hegu (LI 4) dispels excessive heat in the Hand-Yangming Meridian. Jinjin (Extra 10) and Yuye (Extra 9) can activate production of body fluids and check vomiting, especially vomiting due to heat. Needling Fenglong (S 40) strengthens the smooth functioning of the spleen and stomach. Shanzhong (CV 17) regulates qi circulation and resolves sputum. Needling Xuanji (CV 21) and Xiawan (CV 10) conducts the perversive qi downward and activates digestion. Yanglingquan (B 34) and Taichong (Liv 3) are used to bring down the liver and gallbladder qi and stop adverse flow of the liver qi. Needling Pishu (B 20), the Back-Shu point, and Zhangmen (Liv 13), the Front-Mu point, strengthens the spleen qi, leading to normal transportation and transformation. Then digestion occurs and the spleen and stomach work normally.

B. Ear Acupuncture

Main points: Stomach, Liver, Sympathetic Nerve, Subcortex, Ear-Shenmen.

Method: Two or three points are selected each time, with strong stimulation. Needles are retained for twenty to thirty minutes. Treatment is given every day or every other day.

C. Point Injection

Main points: Zusanli (S 36), Zhiyang (GV 9), Lingtai (GV 10).

Method: Select two points alternately for each treatment. Two ml physiological saline is injected into each point once a day.

Remarks

The above treatments may be applied to vomiting due to pregnancy or drug reaction.

Hiccups

Hiccups are due usually to failure of the stomach qi to descend, caused by indigestion, or the adverse flow of the stomach qi, caused by rage. The manifestations are persistent hiccups with a sharp noise. If they occur only occasionally, treatment is unnecessary. If attacks are incessant, treatment aims at relaxing the diaphragm and harmonizing the function of the stomach to bring down the adverse qi. In this case Neiguan (P 6) and Zusanli (S 36) or Juque (CV 14) and Geshu (B 17) are selected.

7. Choking, Food Retardation and Nausea

Choking may occur alone, or it may be the prodrome of food retardation. The two are considered together clinically.

Similar diseases are esophageal cancer, stomach cancer, cardiospasm, phlorus obstruction, esophageal neurosis, etc.

Etiology and Pathology

Choking and food retardation are mostly caused by emotional depression, leading to stagnation of the qi and failure of the body fluids to spread over the body, or by addiction to alcohol and abundant hot food intake, leading to accumulation of heat, which consumes the yin element. The stagnated body fluids from phlegm, together with the excessive heat, obstruct the esophagus. Then difficulty in swallowing occurs, resulting in shortness of qi and blood. A critical condition finally appears, owing to exhaustion of the blood and body fluids and the original qi.

Differentiation

The initial stages are marked by difficulty in swallowing, worsened by emotional depression. Then chest-diaphragm pain, constipation, retardation of food in the esophagus, difficulty in swallowing water, the body all skin and bones, dryness of the throat, dry stool, thin, hesitant pulse, red tongue and little saliva.

Treatment

Method: Remove the obstruction from the chest-diaphragm and harmonize the stomach qi. Reinforcing and reducing methods are used evenly without moxibustion.

Prescription: Geshu (B 17), Juque (CV 14), Neiguan (P 6), Weishu (B 21), Zusanli (S 36).

Explanation: Geshu (B 17) is the influential point of blood, located on the diaphragm. It is selected to promote the circulation of qi and blood, by eliminating the stagnation of heat and sticky phlegm. Juque (CV 14) is the Front-Mu point in the Heart Meridian and Neiguan (P 6) is the connecting point of the pericardium. Since both the Hand-Shaoyin and Hand-Jueyin meridians go along the chest and diaphragm, the two points above are selected for smooth flow of qi in the chest-diaphragm. Needling Weishu (B 21) and Zusanli (S 36) activates the stomach qi and removes obstruction.

Modification: For cases with retardation of food in the esophagus: moxibustion is given to Zhongkui (Extra 26).

For cases with chest and back pain: Neiguan (P 6) and Xinshu (B 15) are added.

For cases with a feeling of diaphragm obstruction: Zhongwan (CV 12) and Daling (P 7) are added.

Remarks

Acupuncture and moxibustion therapy can relieve difficulty in swallowing in esophageal cancer, and it is helpful for cardiospasm and pylorus obstruction.

Nausea

Nausea refers to throwing up food one to two hours after eating, or the food eaten in the morning is vomited in the evening. It is often due to deficiency and cold in the spleen and stomach and lowered functioning of the kidney. Needling is given to Pishu (B 20), Weishu (B 21), Zhongwan (CV 12), Zhangmen (Liv 13), Guanyuan (CV 4), Zusanli (S 36), and Zhongkui (Extra 26) alternately with moxibustion.

8. Diarrhoea

Diarrhoea is caused by dysfunction of the spleen, stomach, and large and small intestines.

It is the manifestation of acute and chronic enteritis and intestinal tuberculosis.

Etiology and Pathology

The condition is classified into acute and chronic categories, described as follows:

(1) Acute diarrhoea: Often due to failure of the stomach and intestines in transportation, transformation and separation of the good from the bad, caused by intake of too much raw and cold or contaminated food or beverage, or affection by exogenous pathogenic agents such as cold, dampness, and summer heat.

(2) Chronic diarrhoea: Due to constantly lowered functioning of the spleen and stomach or deficiency of qi in a protracted illness. The spleen and stomach fail in transportation and transformation, causing troubles in digestion. Sometimes chronic diarrhoea is due to weak functioning of the kidneys and decline of the Gate of Life (area between the kidneys). Food intake can not be digested and diarrhoea follows.

Differentiation

(1) Acute diarrhoea: Marked by sudden onset, with the bowels emptied too often. Cases with excessive damp and cold are manifested by too liquid stool mixed with undigested food, a gurgling sound, abdominal pain, absence of thirst, aversion to cold, slow pulse, smooth white tongue coating. Cases with excessive damp and heat are marked by hot, foul stools, abdominal pain, anus burning, scanty urine, lingering pulse, sticky yellow tongue coating, or fever, thirst, and so on.

(2) Chronic diarrhoea: A prolonged disorder. Sometimes acute diarrhoea develops into chronic. Cases with deficiency in the spleen are manifested by a sallow face, general lassitude, poor appetite, aversion to cold, loose stool, lingering, slow, weak pulse, tender tongue with thin, white coating. Manifestations of cases with deficiency in the kidney are early morning diarrhoea with slight abdominal pain or borborygmus without abdominal pain, chills in the abdomen and lower limbs, deep, thin pulse, pale tongue with white coating.

Treatment

A. Body Acupuncture

(1) Acute diarrhoea

Method: The treatment aims at regulating a smooth flow of qi in the stomach and intestines. For cases with excessive cold, retention of needles is necessary, associated with moxibustion, direct or indirect, with ginger. For cases with excessive heat, the reducing method is employed.

Prescription: Zhongwan (CV 12), Tianshu (S 25), Zusanli (S 36), Yinlingquan (Sp 9).

Explanation: Zhongwan (CV 12), the Front-Mu point of the stomach, and Tianshu (S 25), the Front-Mu point of the large intestine, are selected to harmonize the functions of the stomach and intestines in transportation and transformation, because the Front-Mu point is the place where the qi of the zang-fu organs converge. Zusanli (S 36), the sea point of the stomach, is selected to lower the qi in the stomach and intestines. Since the spleen is united with the stomach in their functional yoke, Yinlingquan (Sp 9) is needled to regulate the spleen qi and make it flow normally. When the vital essence and body fluids spread over the whole body, urine passes freely, retention of dampness is removed and, finally, the bowel movement becomes normal.

(2) Chronic diarrhoea

Method: Strengthen the function of the spleen, stomach and kidney. The reinforcing method is used, often with moxibustion.

Prescription: Pishu (B 20), Zhongwan (CV 12), Zhangmen (Liv 13), Tianshu (S 25), Zusanli (S 36).

Diarrhoea due to deficiency of kidney yang: Mingmen (GV 4), Guanyuan (CV 4).

Explanation: Pishu (B 20) and Zhangmen (Liv 13) are respectively the Back-Shu point and Front-Mu point of the spleen. They are taken together to enhance the function of the spleen. Tianshu (S 25), the Front-Mu point of the large intestine, combined with Zhongwan (CV 12), the Front-Mu point of the stomach, and Zusanli (S 36), the He sea point of the stomach, are needled with the reinforcing method and moxibustion to promote the transporting and transforming functions of the spleen. Moxibustion applied to Mingmen (GV 4) and Guanyuan (CV 4) is to activate the function of the Gate of Life and to warm the spleen and kidneys, making digestion perform normally. It is known as treatment of the root cause.

B. Ear Acupuncture

Main points: Large Intestine, Small Intestine, Stomach, Spleen, Sympathetic Nerve, Ear Shenmen.

Method: Needling with moderate stimulation is given one or two times a day or every other day for chronic cases. Needles are retained for twenty to thirty minutes.

C. Scraping Therapy

It is helpful in mild cases due to summer heat (see "Heat stroke").

Remarks

(1) Diet should be controlled during acute diarrhoea.

(2) Perfusion is advised in dehydration cases.

(3) Dietetic hygiene should be observed in daily life.

9. Dysentery

Dysentery is a common intestinal infectious disease in summer and autumn, marked by abdominal pain, tenesmus, blood and mucus in the stool. It is divided into four types, namely, damp-heat dysentery, damp-cold dysentery, fasting dysentery and relapsing dysentery.

Etiology and Pathology

It is usually caused by affection of damp-heat and intake of contaminated or too much raw and cold food. When the exogenous pathogenic agents and retained food come together, they obstruct the intestines, then the large intestine fails to perform its function in transmission. Furthermore, the confrontation of the dampness with heat and the stagnation of the qi and blood cause injury to the meridians, resulting in mucus and blood in the stool. Preponderance of heat hurts the blood and there is often blood with scant mucus in the stool. Preponderance of dampness damages the qi, causing more mucus with scant blood in the stool. Dysentery due to damp-cold is usually caused by constant deficiency in the spleen and stomach, lowered functioning of the zang-fu organs, affection of exterior cold and accumulation of wind, cold, summer heat and dampness. If there is retention of dampness and heat in the interior and the pathogenic agents stay in the intestines, the spleen and stomach will fail to perform their functions; then dysentery with vomiting will occur and the patient will be unable to eat anything. This is called fasting dysentery. Relapsing dysentery is caused by deficiency of qi in the middle burner and retention of exogenous agents in the intestine. Affection of cold or intake of contaminated food brings it about.

Differentiation

Damp-heat dysentery: Abdominal pain, red and white mucus in the stool, tenesmus, sometimes with a burning sensation in the anus, scant and brownish urine, smooth, rapid pulse, sticky yellow tongue coating, aversion to cold, fever, irascibility, thirst, and so on.

Damp-cold dysentery: Cold, fullness in the chest, lack of taste sense, absence of thirst, sticky white tongue coating, lingering, weak or slow pulse.

Fasting dysentery: Red and white mucus in stool, anorexia, vomiting after eating.

Relapsing dysentery: Persistent recurrence, mild or severe, purulent and bloody stool, abdominal pain, tenesmus, dry or loose stool during remission stage.

Treatment

A. Body Acupuncture

Method: Principal points are in the Hand- and Foot-Yangming meridians, applying the reducing method. For cases of excessive cold, moxibustion is given. For chronic dysentery, treatment of the spleen and kidney is under consideration.

Prescription: Hegu (LI 4), Tianshu (S 25), Shangjuxu (S 37) or Zusanli (S 36).

Damp-heat dysentery: Quchi (LI 11), Neiting (S 44)

Damp-cold dysentery: Zhongwan (CV 12), Qihai (CV 6)

Fasting dysentery: Zhongwan (CV 12), Neiting (S 44)

Relapsing dysentery: Pishu (B 20), Weishu (B 21), Guanyuan (CV 4), Shenshu (B 23)

Explanation: Hegu (LI 4), the He (Sea) point of the Hand-Yangming Meridian, Tianshu (S 25), the Front-Mu point of the large intestine, Shangjuxu (S 37), the inferior He (Sea) point of the large intestine, are used to regulate the qi flow in the large intestine so as to eliminate dampness, because the large intestine is diseased. Quchi (LI 11) and Neiting (S 44) are taken to clear away the dampness and heat form the stomach and intestine. Selection of Zhongwan (CV 12) is to strengthen the stomach qi, remove the dampness and lower the pathogenic factors. Needling Qihai (CV 6) removes the qi stagnation, and moxibustion applied to Qihai (CV 6) warms up the middle burner and dispels cold. Guanyuan (CV 4) and Shenshu (B 23) are used to strengthen the kidney qi and build up body resistance, which is helpful for deficiency and cold in the spleen and kidney.

Modification:

Prolapse of rectum: Moxibustion is added to Baihui (GV 20).

Severe tenesmus: Zhonglüshu (B 29) is added.

B. Ear Acupuncture

See "Diarrhoea."

C. Point Injection

Method: 25 percent solution of glucose or vitamin B_1 (50 mg) is injected into a pair of Tianshu (St 25), 1 ml for each point once a day.

Remarks

(1) Acupuncture-moxibustion therapy is effective for dysentery, but for toxic bacillary dysentery, which is a critical case, comprehensive emergency treatment must be given in time.

(2) Diet control or fasting and isolation of the patient are necessary during the attack.

(3) Do not eat contaminated or bad food.

10. Constipation

Constipation is the inability to empty the bowels over two days, and the waste is hard and solid.

Etiology and Pathology

Constipation can be divided into two categories: excess and deficiency.

(1) Constipation due to excess: Occurs mostly in a person of yang preponderance who prefers peppery or greasy food, causing accumulation of heat in the stomach and intestines. It is also due to pathogenic heat in the interior of the body, impeding body fluids, which leads to dry intestines and stagnation of their qi, or to emotional depression and impediment of the flow of qi, which disturbs the normal dissemination of body fluids and intestinal functions.

(2) Constipation due to deficiency: Often caused by failure to recover qi and blood after an illness or childbirth. Weak and aged people suffer constipation from exhaustion of the qi and blood, resulting in poor functioning and dryness of the intestines. Another cause is deficiency of qi in the lower burner, which makes cold accumulate. The qi passage of the intestines is blocked and constipation occurs.

Differentiation

(1) Constipation due to excess: It is marked by fewer and difficult bowel movements, usually once in three to five days or even longer. If it is due to accumulation of excessive pathogenic heat, the manifestations are body heat, thirst, foul breath, preference for cold, smooth pulse, dry yellow tongue coating. Cases of stagnation of qi are manifested by fullness and distension or pain in the hypochondriac region and abdomen, frequent sighing, poor appetite, taut pulse, thin, sticky tongue coating.

(2) Constipation due to deficiency: For cases of deficiency of the qi and blood it is manifested by pallor, pale lips and nails, dizziness and vertigo, general lassitude, pale tongue with thin coating, weak, thin pulse. Accumulation of cold leads to abdominal pain, cold sensation in the abdomen, preference for warmth and dislike of cold, deep, slow pulse, pale tongue with moist white coating.

Treatment

A. Body Acupuncture

Method: Main points are the Back-Shu point, the Front-Mu point and the inferior He (Sea) point of the Large Intestine Meridian. The reducing method is used for constipation due to excess and the reinforcing method for constipation due to deficiency. For constipation due to cold, moxibustion is given as well.

Prescription: Dachangshu (B 25), Tianshu (S 25), Zhigou (TE 6), Shangjuxu (S 37).

Accumulation of heat: Hegu (LI 4), Quchi (LI 11).

Stagnation of qi: Zhongwan (CV 12), Xingjian (Liv 2).

Deficiency of qi and blood: Pishu (B 20), Weishu (B 21).

Constipation due to cold: Moxibustion applied to Shenque (CV 8) and Qihai (CV 6).

Explanation: Constipation varies as to cause, yet it is always a dysfunctioning of the large intestine in transmission. Therefore, Dachangshu (B 25) and Tianshu (S 25), the Back-Shu point and the Front-Mu point of the Large Intestine Meridian are selected, combined with Shangjuxu (S 37), the inferior He (Sea) point of the Large Intestine Meridian, to strengthen the flow of qi in the large intestine until it finally functions normally. Zhigou (TE 6) removes obstruction in the triple burners for normal functioning of the large intestine. Quchi (LI 11) and Hegu (LI 4) promote downward flow of qi in the large intestine and eliminate excessive heat. Zhongwan (CV 12), the influential point of the fu organs, is used to bring a downward flow of qi in the large intestine. The reducing method is applied to Xingjian (Liv 2) to soothe the liver qi. For cases with depression of the liver qi, needling Pishu (B 20) and Weishu (B 21) with the reinforcing method helps strengthen the function of the middle burner. When qi in the spleen and stomach is flourishing, more blood is produced. This is considered the treatment for the root cause of constipation. Moxibustion applied to Qihai (CV 6) and Shenque (CV 8) warms up the triple burners and removes cold.

B. Ear Acupuncture

Main points: Lower portion of rectum, Large Intestine, Subcortex.

Method: Needling is given with moderate, intermittent stimulation. Needles are retained for ten to twenty minutes.

Remarks

The patient should eat more vegetables and maintain regular bowel movements.

11. Prolapse of Rectum

Prolapse of rectum refers to a condition of protrusion of the rectal mucus membrane through the anus to varying degree, often seen in children, the aged and women of multiple parturition.

Etiology and Pathology

Prolapse of rectum is mostly caused by prolonged diarrhoea, chronic dysentery, and weak constitution after an attack of a severe disease or frequent childbirth, all of which result in the loss of qi in the middle burner and failure of its function to keep the organs in normal position.

Differentiation

The illness progresses slowly. At first one feels only a distending and bearing-down sensation of the anus during bowel movements, and the prolapsed rectum returns to its normal position. But if the condition is prolonged, as often occurs when the patient is overtired, the prolapsed rectum no longer returns automatically to its normal position and must be helped with one's fingers. The condition is usually marked by general lassitude, unhealthy complexion, dizziness, palpitation, weak, thin pulse, pale tongue with white coating.

Treatment

A. Body Acupuncture

Method: Principal points are in the Governor Vessel Meridian. Needling is the reinforcing method. Moxibustion is applicable.

Prescription: Baihui (GV 20), Changqiang (GV 1), Dachangshu (B 25).

Explanation: The rectum is the end of the large intestine. Needling Dachangshu (B 25) with the reinforcing method strengthens the vital function of the large intestine. Baihui (GV 20), the crossing point of the Governor Vessel Meridian and the three yang meridians, pertaining to yang, is controlled by the Governor Vessel Meridian, so moxibustion applied to Baihui (GV 20) makes the yang flourish and restores the rectunis lifting ability. Changqiang (GV 1) is located in one of the collaterals of the Governor Vessel Meridian close to the anus. Needling the point strengthens the contractive function of the anus. The three points prescribed above are used to make the sinking qi rise.

Modification: Qihai (CV 6), Zusanli (S 36), Shenshu (B 23), Pishu (B 20).

B. Picking Therapy

Any spot in the longitudinal line 1 to 1.5 cun lateral to the middle line of the spine between the third lumbar vertebra and second sacral vertebra.

C. Ear Acupuncture

Main points: Lower portion of rectum, Subcortex, Ear Shenmen.

Method: Needling is given once a day with moderate stimulation. Needles are retained for thirty minutes.

Remarks

Medication is advisable for cases with prolapse of rectum due to weak constitution.

12. Retention of Urine

Difficulty in urination is considered a mild case; complete retention of urine is a serious condition.

Etiology and Pathology

Retention of urine indicates the lesion is in the urinary bladder, caused by disturbance in the function of the urinary bladder due to injury to the kidney qi, consumption of qi and blood, and lowered functioning of the Gate of Life. It is also due to excessive dampness and heat in the middle burner, which goes down to the urinary bladder and blocks the qi, or to traumatic injuries or a surgical operation on the lower abdomen, which damages the qi passage of the urinary bladder.

Differentiation

(1) Insufficiency of kidney qi: Marked by dribbling urination, general lassitude, pallor, weakness in the lumbar region and knees, pale tongue, deep, thin pulse, especially weak in the ulnar region.

(2) Downward flow of dampness and heat: Manifested by scant and brown urine or complete retention of urine, distended sensation in the lower abdomen, thirst, red tongue with yellow coating, rapid pulse.

(3) Traumatic injury: Main complaints are difficulty in urination and fullness and distended sensation in lower abdomen, found in cases having a history of traumatic injuries or surgical operation.

Treatment

A. Body Acupuncture

a. Insufficiency of kidney qi

Method: Main points are in the Foot-Shaoyin Meridian, supplemented by Back-Shu points in the Urinary-bladder Meridian. The reinforcing method and/or moxibustion is used.

Prescription: Yingu (K 10), Shenshu (B 23), Sanjiaoshu (B 22), Qihai (CV 6), Weiyang (B 39).

Explanation: It is of primary importance to replenish the kidney qi in cases of insufficiency of kidney qi and lowered functioning of the Gate of Life. Yingu (K 10), the He (Sea) point of the Kidney Meridian, is selected with Shenshu (B 23) to strengthen the kidney qi. Insufficient kidney qi leads to disturbance in the function of the triple burners. Sanjiaoshu (B 22) and Weiyang (B 39), the inferior He (Sea) points of the triple burners, are selected to regulate the flow of qi. Moxibustion applied to Qihai (CV 6) warms up the lower burner and strengthen its function. All the treatments aim at strengthening the kidney qi and regulating the function of the triple burners to make normal urination possible.

b. Downward flow of damp heat

Method: Main points are in the Foot-Taiyin Meridian. The reducing method is used without moxibustion.

Prescription: Sanyinjiao (Sp 6), Yinlingquan (Sp 9), Pangguangshu (B 28), Zhongji (CV 3).

Explanation: This disease is due mainly to damp-heat in the spleen channel flowing downward to the urinary bladder. Yinlingquan (Sp 9), the He (Sea) point of the Foot-Taiyin Meridian, is used with Sanyinjiao (Sp 6) to promote qi circulation in the spleen meridian. The urinary bladder controls the body's water metabolism. When dampness and heat accumulate in it, the urinary bladder fails to work well. Therefore, Pangguangshu (B 28) and Zhongji (CV 3), the Front-Mu points of the urinary bladder, are selected to normalize the water metabolism in the urinary bladder and drive away the damp heat.

c. Traumatic injury

Method: Regulation of qi flow in the urinary bladder is the aim of treatment. Moxibustion is applied according to one's condition.

Prescription: Zhongji (CV 3) and Sanyinjiao (Sp 6).

Explanation: The traumatic injury or surgical operation may block the qi passage of the urinary bladder and cause retention of urine. Selection of Zhongji (CV 3), the Front-Mu point of the urinary bladder, with Sanyinjiao (Sp 6), where the three yin meridians converge, promotes a smooth flow of the qi in the urinary bladder and removes retention of urine.

B. Ear Acupuncture

Main points: Kidney, Urinary Bladder, Sympathetic Nerve, External Genitalia, Subcortex.

Method: Two to four points are selected for each treatment with moderate or strong stimulation. Needles are retained for twenty to thirty minutes.

C. Electroacupuncture

A pair of Weidao (G 28) points are needled to a depth of about two to three cun with the tip of the needles going towards Qugu (CV 2). Electricity is on for fifteen to thirty minutes.

Remarks

(1) When the urinary bladder is overfull, shallow or oblique puncture on the points of the lower abdomen is advisable. Never use deep and perpendicular puncture.

(2) Proper measures must be taken for cases due to mechanical obstruction or nervous injury. Identify the causative factors.

13. Urination Disturbance

Urination disturbance refers to frequent urination and slow, painful discharge of urine. It is usually classified into five kinds: Dysfunction of the urinary bladder, urolithiasis, hematuria, chyluria and overstrain.

The condition includes infection and calculi in the urinary tract.

Etiology and Pathology

Urination disturbance is mainly caused by heat in the urinary bladder. Accumulation of dampness and heat in the urinary bladder damages the blood vessels, resulting in hematuria with urethral pain. Urolithiasis is due to accumulation of heat in the lower buner. The urine is heated and the turbid part turns into gravel. When there is malfunction of the urinary bladder, impeding normal production of urine, chyluria occurs. Sometimes difficulty in urination is caused by a painful distension of the lower abdomen due to injury to the liver caused by rage. Excessive fire rushes to the urinary bladder and causes its dysfunction. Intemperance in sexual life is another reason for dysuria. Because exhaustion of the kidney qi causes deficiency in the kidney or spleen, that in turn affects the function of the urianry bladder.

Differentiation

The manifestations of the disease are urethral pain when passing water, dribbling urination or complete retention of urine when there is a distension of the lower abdomen, sudden pain in the lumbar region and hematuria, or urine containing gravel, or turbid, greasy urine.

Treatment

A. Body Acupuncture

Method: Treatment aims at promoting smooth flow of the qi in the urinary bladder and normal flow of urine and pain killing. The reducing method or a half reinforcing, half reducing method is used.

Prescription: Pangguangshu (B 28), Zhongji (CV 3), Yinlingquan (G 34), Xingjian (Liv 2), Taixi (K 3).

Explanation: The lesion of the disease is in the urinary bladder. Pangguangshu (B 28) and Zhongji (CV 3) are selected to restore the normal function of the urinary bladder. Selection of Yinlingquan (G 34), the He (Sea) point of the Spleen Meridian, is for smooth flow of urine and removal of pain, for pain is caused by obstruction. The Liver Meridian curves around the genital organs, therefore Xingjian (Liv 2), the Xing (Spring) point of the Liver Meridian, is used to reduce the fire in the Liver Meridian and stop pain. Taixi (K 3), the Yuan (Source) point of the Kidney Meridian, is taken to purge the water in the kidney.

Modifications:

Hematuria: Xuehai (Sp 10) and Sanyinjiao (Sp 6) are added.

Turbid, greasy urine: Shenshu (B 23) and Zhaohai (K 6) are added.

Distension pain of the lower abdomen: Ququan (Liv 8) is added.

Urine containing gravel: Weiyang (B 39) and Rangu (K 2) are added.

Overstrain: Xingjian (Liv 2) is left out and moxibustion is applied to Baihui (GV 20) and Qihai (CV 6).

B. Ear Acupuncture

Main points: Urinary Bladder, Kidney, Sympathetic Nerve, Occiput, Adrenal.

Method: Two to four points are selected for each treatment. Needles are retained for twenty to thirty minutes. Manipulate the needles once or twice. Points selected above are effective for cystitis. For pyelonephritis it is advisable to add Liver and Endocrine.

C. Electroacupuncture

Main points: Shenshu (B 23) and Sanyinjiao (Sp 6).

Method: The current is on for five to ten minutes. Strong stimulation with high-frequency pulse is used. The points given above are also used for treating renal colic.

Remarks

(1) Acupuncture-moxibustion therapy can relieve irritant symptoms of urinary tract infection and alleviate pain of renal colic caused by renal calculi.

(2) Women should be concerned with hygiene during menstruation and childbirth to avoid urinary tract infection.

(3) A patient with urinary calculi should drink plenty of water and do jumping exercises to help excretion of stones.

14. Seminal Emission

Seminal emission may be nocturnal (with dreams) or involuntary. In general, seminal emission once a week is considered normal for unmarried young men. Treatment is unnecessary.

Etiology and Pathology

Seminal emission is due mostly to anxiety or sexual indulgence, resulting in consumption of the vital essence of the heart and lack of communication between heart and kidney, when the heart fire cannot descend to the kidney and the kidney water cannot ascend to the heart. Deficiency of kidney water and blazing fire in the heart and kidney disturbs the seminal bank and causes emission. Addiction to alcohol and greasy food makes the dampness and heat flow downward, which leads to emission. Intermittent spermatorrhea exhausts the kidney qi, which fails to control emission, often causing involuntary emission.

Differentiation

Nocturnal emission usually occurs during dreaming when the penis tends to erect. A prolonged case is often associated with dizziness, listlessness, ringing in the ears, and pain in the lumbar region.

Involuntary emission occurs anytime when the sexual desire comes. The manifestations are emaciation, thin, soft pulse, palpitation, impotence.

Treatment

A. Body Acupuncture

Method: For nocturnal emission, treatment aims at harmonizing the relationship between the heart and the kidney. Puncturing is given with half reinforcing, half reducing methods. For involuntary emission, it is essential to strengthen the kidney function. The reinforcing method and/or moxibustion is used.

Prescription: Guanyuan (CV 4), Dahe (K 12), Zhishi (G 52).

Nocturnal emission: Xinshu (B 15), Shenmen (H 7), Neiguan (P 6).

Involuntary emission: Shenshu (B 23), Taixi (K 3), Zusanli (S 36).

Explanation: Guanyuan (CV 4), the juncture of the three foot yin meridians and the Conception Vessel Meridian and the base of the body's primary qi, is used to activate the kidney qi. Guanyuan (CV 4), combined with Zhishi (G 52) and Dahe (K 12), is selected to strengthen the guard of the sperm bank. For nocturnal emission, Xinshu (B 15), Shenmen (H 7) and Neiguan (P 6) are taken to cause the heart fire to descend and harmonize the relationship between the heart and kidney. For involuntary emission, Shenshu (B 23) and Taixi (K 3) are used to strengthen the kidney; replenish the resource of transformation of blood and qi by taking Zusanli (S 36).

B. Point Injection

Main points: Guanyuan (CV 4) and Zhongji (CV 3).

Method: A small amount of vitamin B_1 solution or Chinese angelica solution is injected into Guanyuan (CV 4) and Zhongji (CV 3). When the syringe needle is inserted into the point and the needling sensation reaches the anterior pubic region, the solution is put into the point. Treatment is given every other day. Ten times constitutes a treatment course.

C. Ear Acupuncture

Main points: Essence Palace, Endocrine, Ear Shenmen, Liver, Kidney.

Method: Two to four points are punctured for each treatment. Needles are retained for ten to thirty minutes or embedded for three to five days.

D. Cutaneous Needling

Tapping is applied to the lumborsacral region and the inner sides of the lower limbs for fifteen minutes. Treatment is given every day or every other day.

Remarks

(1) Seminal emission is usually a functional disorder; it should not cause much worry.

(2) If it is caused by some organic disease, the primary disease must be cured simultaneously.

15. Impotence

Etiology and Pathology

Impotence is usually caused by early marriage and sexual indulgence and masturbation in adolescence, resulting in weakness of the Gate of Life and loss of the kidney qi. Fear may also injure the kidney function and lead to impotence.

Differentiation

Impotence is characterized by inability of the penis to erect, often associated with dizziness and vertigo, pallor, listlessness, weakness and pain in the lower back and legs, thin, weak pulse.

Treatment

A. Body Acupuncture

Method: Strengthening the kidney qi is the aim of treatment. The reinforcing method and/or moxibustion is used.

Prescription: Shenshu (B 23), Mingmen (GV 4), Sanyinjiao (Sp 6), Guanyuan (CV 4).

Explanation: This disease results from exhaustion of the kidney qi, so Shenshu (B 23), Mingmen (GV 4) and Sanyinjiao (Sp 6) are applied to intensify the kidney function. Needling Guanyuan (CV 4), where the primary is stored, with the reinforcing method can fill the primary qi and activate the function of the kidney meridian.

B. Electroacupuncture

Main points: a. Baliao (B 31-34) and Rangu (K 2). b. Guanyuan (CV 4) and Sanyinjiao (Sp 6).

Method: Two groups of points can be used alternately with low-frequency pulse and current connected for three to five minutes.

C. Ear Acupuncture

Main points: Essence Palace, External Genitalia, Testis, Endocrine.

Method: Same as for seminal emission.

D. Point Injection

Main points: Guanyuan (CV 4), Zhongji (CV 3), Shenshu (B 23).

Method: Inject 50 mg vitamin B_1 solution or 5 mg *Testosterone Propionte* into the three points in turn. The treatment interval is two to three days. Four treatments constitute a course.

Remarks

(1) Impotence is often a functional disturbance. Advise the patient not to worry too much about it.

(2) During the course of treatment suspend sexual activity.

16. Pulmonary Tuberculosis

Pulmonary tuberculosis is a chronic consumptive and infectious disease caused by infection of the bacillus tubercle (ancient people called it "tuberculous insect") when body resistance is low or after frequent contact with a TB patient.

It is called "bone steaming" and "infectious corpse" in ancient Chinese medical literature.

Etiology and Pathology

The causative agents of this disease include an external factor, the infection of bacillus tubercle, and an internal factor, low body resistance. The lesion is located in the lungs. In the initial stages consumption of the vital essence of the lungs and impairment of the lungs by fire appear. If the case is prolonged, the spleen and kidney will be injured, leading to exhaustion of the primary qi and deficiency of both yin and yang.

Differentiation

The manifestations of the disease are cough, hectic fever, night sweating, hemoptysis, emaciation. In general, deficiency of yin is often seen clinically. The early stages are characterized by intermittent cough, lassitude, poor appetite, gradual emaciation, insidious chest pain, bloody sputum and dry cough with expectoration of less sputum, afternoon fever, malar flush, nocturnal sweating, hemoptysis in large amount, irascibility, insomnia, seminal emission in men, amenorrhea in women, red tongue, thin, rapid pulse. Manifestations of a prolonged case are emaciation, hoarseness of voice, loose stool, swollen face and limbs, smooth dark-red tongue, and fading pulse, denoting a critical condition.

Treatment

A. Body Acupuncture

Method: Main points are in the Hand-Taiyin Meridian and the Back-Shu points. Acupuncture is often given for cases with deficiency of yin. Moxibustion is mostly given to cases with deficiency of yang.

Prescription: Chize (L 5), Feishu (B 13), Gaohuangshu (B 43), Dazhui (GV 14), Sanyinjiao (Sp 6), Taixi (K 3).

Explanation: Chize (L 5), the He (Sea) point of the Lung Meridian, and Feishu (B 13) clear out excessive heat in the Lung Meridian. Gaohuangshu (B 43) and Dazhui (GV 14), the empirical points in treatment of pulmonary tuberculosis, and Dazhui (GV 14) intensify the lung qi and the primary qi. Sanyinjiao (Sp 6) strengthens the spleen function and activates the lung qi. Taixi (K 3), the Yuan (Source) point of the Kidney Meridian, promotes the production of kidney water and suppresses fire.

Modification:

Hectic fever: Yuji (L 10), Laogong (P 8) and Taixi (K 3) are added.

Night sweating: Yinxi (H 6) and Fuliu (K 7) are added.

Hemoptysis: Zhongfu (L 1), Kongzui (L 6) and Geshu (B 17) are added.

Hoarseness of voice: Taiyuan (L 9) and Tianding (LI 17) are added.

Seminal emission: Zhishi (B 52), Guanyuan (CV 4) and Sanyinjiao (Sp 6) are added.

Amenorrhea: Xuehai (Sp 10) and Diji (Sp 8) are added.

When yang deficiency occurs, add Pishu (B 20), Shenshu (B 23) and Guanyuan (CV 4); scarring moxibustion is also applied to the Back-Shu points.

B. Point Injection

Main points: Zhongfu (L 1), Feishu (B 13), and Dazhui (GV 14), associated with Gaohuang (B 43), Quchi (LI 11), and Zusanli (S 36).

Method: Vitamin B_1 solution (100 mg) or streptomycin solution (0.2 g) is injected into each point. Two or three points are selected for each treatment.

Remarks

Administer anti-TB herbs simultaneously with acupuncture-moxibustion therapy to strengthen the results.

17. Insomnia and Amnesia

Insomnia is also known as fail to sleep in ancient Chinese medical literature. It is habitual inability to fall asleep or restless sleep.

Etiology and Pathology

There are various causes for insomnia, such as mental anxiety and strain, impairment of the heart and spleen, sexual indulgence resulting in injury to the kidney and disharmony between the heart and kidney, deficiency of qi in the heart and gallbladder, and mental depression, leading to hyperactive yang of the liver and disorder of the stomach.

Differentiation

Difficulty in falling asleep is manifested in various ways: Inability to sleep upon going to bed, waking up easily and not being able to fall asleep again, restless sleep, and inability to fall asleep at all. Different manifestations indicate different causes. For example, insomnia due to deficiency in the heart and spleen is manifestated by dream-distured sleep, palpitation, amnesia, sweating, thin, weak pulse. Insomnia due to deficiency in the kidney is manifested by vertigo, tinnitus, nocturnal emission, low back pain, red tongue, thin, rapid pulse. Insomnia due to deficiency in the kidney is manifested by vertigo, tinnitus, nocturnal emission, low back pain, red tongue, thin, rapid pulse. Insomnia due to deficiency of qi in the heart and gallbladder often produces palpitation, dreams in sleep, susceptibility to fright, pale tongue, taut, thin pulse. Insomnia due to mental depression resulting from disturbance of the liver yang may take the form of irascibility, dizziness, headache, distension pain in the hypochondriac region, taut pulse. Insomnia caused by disorder of the qi in the stomach produces a suffocating feeling in the epigastric region, belching or distension pain in the epigastrium and abdomen, thick, sticky tongue coating, smooth pulse.

Treatment

A. Body Acupuncture

Method: Tranquilizing the mind is the treatment principle. The Yuan (Source) points or Back-Shu points of the affected meridians are selected alternately according to differentiation of syndromes. The reinforcing or half reinforcing, half reducing method and/or moxibustion is used.

Prescription: Shenmen (H 7) and Sanyinjiao (S 6).

Modification:

Deficiency of qi in the heart and spleen: Xinshu (B 15), Jueyinshu (B 14) and Pishu (B 20) are added.

Hypofunction of the kidney: Xinshu (B 15), Shenshu (B 23) and Taixi (K 3) are added.

Deficiency of qi in the heart and gallbladder: Xinshu (B 15), Danshu (B 19), Daling (P 7) and Qiuxu (G 40) are added.

Upward disturbance of the liver yang: Ganshu (B 18), Jianshi (P 5) and Taichong (Liv 3) are added.

Disharmony of the spleen and stomach: Weishu (B 21) and Zusanli (S 36) are added.

Explanation: The Yuan (Source) point of the Heart Meridian is used to calm the mind. Sanyinjiao (Sp 6) is taken to restore the balance of yin and yang in the three foot-yin meridians. The Yuan (Source) points of the involved meridian or the Back-Shu points are selected in view of different causes. For instance, the reinforcing method or moxibustion applied to Xinshu (B 15) and Pishu (B 20) strengthens the function of the heart and spleen. Xinshu (B 15) and Shenshu (B 23) are employed to activate the heart and kidney, enabling the kidney water to irrigate the heart and the heart fire to warm the kidney. For cases with mental restlessness resulting from hyperactive yang of the liver, Ganshu (B 18) and Taichong (Liv 3) are chosen to reduce the liver. Weishu (B 21) and Zusanli (S 36) are used to regulate the stomach, because disorder of the stomach can cause nocturnal restlessness.

B. Ear Acupuncture

Main points: Subcortex, Sympathetic Nerve, Heart, Spleen, Kidney, Endocrine, Ear Shenmen.

Method: Two or three points are selected for each treatment with moderate stimulations. Needles are retained for twenty minutes.

Amnesia

Amnesia refers to loss of memory, either in part or completely. It is usually due to dysfunction of the reservoir of medulla or the brain and deprivation of blood of the heart and essence of the kidney.

Treatment

Baihui (GV 20), Yintang (Extra 1), Xinshu (B 15), Pishu (B 20), Shenshu (B 23), Zhaohai (K 6), Xuanzhong (G 39) and Zusanli (S 36) are selected. Needling is done with the reinforcing method.

18. Palpitation of the Heart

Palpitation of the heart refers to irregular heartbeat and susceptibility to fright, usually induced by emotional disturbance or overexertion. In severe cases there may be continuous and uncontrollable violent throbbing of the heart.

Etiology and Pathology

Palpitation usually occurs in someone with a weak constitution and deficiency of qi in the heart when he is frightened or angry or encounters thrilling or dangerous conditions. It is stated in "Candid Question,"* "Fright leads to disturbance of the mind and the configurative force and failure to make decisions." All this infers disturbed flow of qi. Other reasons for palpitation are blood deficiency in the heart, fire flaring due to yin deficiency, hypoactivity of the heart, upward disturbance of phlegm heat.

Differentiation

Palpitation is usually marked by paroxysm, susceptibility to fright, restlessness, dream-disturbed sleep, weak, taut pulse, normal tongue coating. Cases with blood deficiency of the heart may show pallor, vertigo, disturbed sleep, pale tongue, weak, thin pulse. Cases with fire flaring due to yin deficiency may produce distress, insomnia, dizziness, tinnitus, red tongue, thin, rapid pulse. Cases with interior retention of fluid due

*The first part of *Inner Classic of the Yellow Sovereign.*

to hypoactivity of the heart may manifest fullness in the chest and epigastrium, lassitude, cold extremities, aversion to cold, white tongue coating, taut, smooth pulse. Cases with upward disturbance of phlegm heat may manifest irritability and restlessness, dream-disturbed sleep, yellow tongue coating, smooth, rapid pulse.

Treatment

A. Body Acupuncture

Method: Main points are in the Hand-Shaoyin and Foot-Yueyin meridians, combined with the Back-Shu points. Needling is done with the half reinforcing, half reducing method.

Prescription: Jianshi (P 5), Shenmen (H 7), Xinshu (B 15), Juque (CV 14).

Modification:

Blood deficiency of the heart: Geshu (B 17), Pishu (B 20) and Zusanli (S 36) are added.

Fire flaring due to yin deficiency: Jueyinshu (B 14), Shenshu (B 23) and Taixi (L 3) are added.

Interior retention of fluid: Pishu (B 20), Sanjiaoshu (B 22) and Qihaishu (B 24) are added.

Upward disturbance of phlegm heat: Feishu (B 13), Chize (L 5) and Fenglong (S 40) are added.

Explanation: Treatment aims at calming the mind and stopping fright. Shenmen (H 7), the Yuan (Source) point of the Heart Meridian, and Xinshu (B 15), the Back-Shu point of the Heart Meridian are taken with Juque (CV 14), the Front-Mu point of the Heart Meridian, and Jianshi (P 5), the Jing (River) point of the Pericardium Meridian to regulate the passage of qi of the heart, thus calming the mind and checking fright. In cases of blood deficiency, Geshu (B 17), the influential point dominating blood, Pishu (B 20) and Zusanli (S 36) strengthen the constitution. Deficiency of yin and fire flaring indicate insufficient vital essence in the kidney, therefore Shenshu (B 23), Taixi (K 3), and Jueyinshu (B 14) are used to refresh the yin of the kidney. Pishu (B 20), Sanjiaoshu (B 22) and Qihaishu (B 24) are selected to activate the flow of qi and remove the interior retention of harmful fluid. For upward disturbance of phlegm and heat, Feishu (B 13), Chize (L 5) and Fenglong (S 40) are employed to resolve phlegm and clear off heat so that the qi in the lungs is able to descend and palpitation stops.

B. Ear Acupuncture

Main points: Heart, Subcortex, Sympathetic Nerve, Ear Shenmen.

Method: Two or three points are used for each treatment. Needling is done with mild twirling. Needles are retained for fifteen minutes.

Vigorous palpitation: It is characterized by frequent, uncontrollable palpitation, a suffocating feeling in the chest and paroxysmal heart pain in severe cases.

Prescription: Xinshu (B 15), Jueyinshu (B 14), Ximen (P 4), Neiguan (P 6), Tongli (H 5), Taichong (Liv 3), Taixi (K 3).

Method: The reinforcing method is usually used.

19. Depressive and Manic Mental Disorders

Both depressive and manic mental disorders are caused by imbalance of yin and yang and failure of the mind to control itself, resulting from mental depression, melancholy, anxiety and exasperation, which elicit fire and cause formation of phlegm. Manic and depressive mental disorders both pertain to excess type.

Etiology and Pathology

(1) Depressive mental disorder

It is usually due to melancholy, anxiety and mental depression, leading to dysfunction of the liver in free movement of the qi. When the spleen qi fails to work properly, phlegm is formed by the stagnated body fluid. When the phlegm goes upward perversely and causes derangement of the mind, depressive mental disorder results.

(2) Manic mental disorder

It is due mainly to one's desires' not being satisfied, abundant fire in the liver and stomach, and upward disturbance of the phlegm, which lead to mental disturbance and failure of the mind to control itself.

Differentiation

(1) Depressive mental disorder is characterized by muteness and dullness, mental depression, apathy, paraphasia, paraphrenia, foolish fancies, suspicion and susceptibility to fright, poor appetite, greasy yellow tongue coating, taut and thin or smooth pulse.

(2) Manic mental disorder is manifested by sudden onset, shouting and yelling, restlessness, preceded by irritability, headache, insomnia, flushed face, redness of the eyes, smashing things, hurting oneself, hitting, unusual strength, no desire to eat, deep-red tongue with sticky yellow coating, taut, smooth pulse.

Treatment

A. Body Acupuncture

a. Depressive mental disorder

Method: The Back-Shu points are mainly selected, coordinated with the Yuan (Source) points and connecting points. Needling is given with the half reinforcing, half reducing method.

Prescription: Xinshu (B 15), Ganshu (B 18), Pishu (B 20), Shenmen (H 7), Fenglong (S 40).

Explanation: As the disorder chiefly results from the depression of qi and accumulation of phlegm in the heart and spleen, Xinshu (B 15), Ganshu (B 18) and Pishu (B 20) are used to open the aperture of the heart blocked by the phlegm, ease the liver and strengthen the function of the spleen, while Shenmen (H 7) and Fenglong (S 40) are taken to resolve phlegm and tranquilize the mind.

b. Manic mental disorder

Method: Main points are in the Governor Vessel Meridian, combined with some others to clear off phlegm fire. Needling is given with the reducing method.

Prescription: Dazhui (GV 14), Fengfu (GV 16), Shuigou (GV 26), Neiguan (P 6), Fenglong (S 40).

Explanation: Dazhui (GV 14) and Shuigou (GV 26) are used in combination to dispel the pathogenic factors from the brain. Fengfu (GV 16) is prescribed according to the theory in the "Treatise on the Reservoir, Miraculous Pivot"* that "the brain is the reservoir of medulla; its vital energy infuses downward into point Fengfu." A combination of Neiguan (P 6) and Fenglong (S 40) is prescribed for regulating the stomach and lowering the phlegm, so that the mind can be controlled, thus stopping the manic mental disorder.

B. Electroacupuncture

Main points: Group 1: Shuigou (GV 26), Baihui (GV 20).
Group 2: Dazhui (GV 14), Fengfu (GV 16) towards Yamen (GV 15).

Method: One group is selected for each treatment. Electric stimulation is given for fifteen to twenty minutes after the insertion of needles. Wave forms are based on the individual case. Strong stimulation is advisable for manic mental disorder and short, intermittent and strong stimulation for depressive mental disorder.

C. Point Injection

Main points: Xinshu (B 15), Geshu (B 17), Jianshi (P 5), Zusanli (S 36), Sanyinjiao (Sp 6).

Method: A solution made of 25 to 50 mg chlorpromazine is injected into one or alternately two of the selected points once a day for manic disorder.

D. Ear Acupuncture

Main points: Subcortex, Heart, Kidney, Occiput, Forehead.

Method: Three or four points are punctured for each treatment. Needles are retained for thirty minutes. Body acupuncture may also be applied in combination.

Remarks

During treatment, nursing care should be strengthened and ideological education be performed attentively.

20. Epilepsy

Epilepsy is a paroxysmal disease of the brain that causes sudden attacks of uncontrolled violent movement and loss of consciousness, denoting psychic or sensory disturbances. After revival the patient becomes normal.

Etiology and Pathology

The causative factor is upward disturbance of phlegm, resulting in a loss of consciousness. Some cases are genetic, occurring in childhood. Some are induced by mental irritation or other affections. Dysfunction of the heart, kidney, liver and spleen can lead to temporary derangement of yin and yang. When the pathogenic agents of yang nature rises, interior wind is stirred up and phlegm confuses the mind. Then epilepsy attacks suddenly.

Differentiation

Epilepsy usually pertains to excess, but a relapse or a prolonged case may develop into a deficiency type. There may be vertigo, stuffiness in the chest or lassitude before

---

*The second part of *Inner Classic of the Yellow Sovereign.*

onset, followed by sudden loss of consciousness or clenched jaws, eyes staring upward, convulsion of the limbs, slobbering or incontinence of feces and urine. After the attack dizziness, general weakness of the limbs, general lassitude, thin, sticky tongue coating, taut, smooth pulse may appear. In prolonged cases the pulse is thin and soft.

Treatment

A. Body Acupuncture

Method: Main points are in Conception Vessel and Governor Vessel meridians, coordinated with points that can remove phlegm and unconsciousness.

Prescription: Jiuwei (CV 15), Dazhui (GV 14), Yaoqi (Extra 20), Jianshi (P 5), Fenglong (S 40).

Explanation: Treatment aims at resolving phlegm and checking pathogenic wind. Jiuwei (CV 15), the connecting point of the Conception Vessel Meridian, and Dazhui (GV 14), the crossing point of the six yang meridians, are used to regulate yin and yang. Fenglong (S 40) activates the function of the spleen and stomach in transportation and transformation so as to resolve phlegm and stop phlegm formation. Jianshi (P 5) regulates the qi of the Pericardium Meridian for resuscitation. Yaoqi (Extra 20), as an empirical point, combined with Jiuwei (CV 15) is most helpful.

B. Suture-embedding Therapy

Main points: Dazhui (GV 14), Yaoqi (Extra 20), Jiuwei (CV 15).

Secondary points: Yiming (Extra 7), Shenmen (H 7).

Method: Two or Three points are embedded with suture for each treatment. Then interval of treatment is twenty days. Commonly used points and secondary points may be used alternately.

C. Point Injection

Main points: Zusanli (S 36), Neiguan (P 6), Dazhui (GV 14), Fengchi (G 20).

Method: A solution of vitamin B_1 (100 mg) or vitamin B_{12} (0.5 to 1 mg) is taken. Inject 0.5 ml solution into the selected point. Two or three points are used for each treatment.

D. Ear Acupuncture

Main points: Stomach, Subcortex, Ear Shenmen, Occiput, Heart.

Method: Needles are retained for twenty to thirty minutes and twirled intermittently, or ear needles are embedded for three to seven days. Three to five points are taken for each treatment.

Remarks

For cases caused by other affections, the case history should be investigated and special examinations taken to make a correct diagnosis. Treat the primary affections first.

21. Vertigo

Vertigo in traditional Chinese medicine refers to blurring of vision and dizziness in the head. In mild cases vertigo will be suppressed very soon after lying down and closing the eyes. In severe cases the patient may have the sensation of being in a boat or in a running vehicle, rising, falling and turning around. Vertigo may occur in hypertension, arteriosclerosis, anemia, neurosis, otogenic disorder and tumour in the head.

Etiology and Pathology

Vertiago is related to a weak constitution, debility after an illness, melancholy, anxiety, exasperation, and intake of greasy food. A detailed analysis shows it may result from deficiency of yang, weakness of qi, and failure of the primary qi to reach the brain, or from yin deficiency of the kidney, leading to a weak yang floating upward. It may also be due to excessive dampness in the body and too much greasy food, which produce phlegm, which blocks fire.

Differentiation

The clinical manifestations are dizziness, blurring of vision, frequent nausea, failure to stand firmly. If weakness of the limbs, pallor, palpitation, sleeplessness, aversion to cold, lying with the body curled, thin, weak pulse appear, it indicates deficiency of qi and blood. Low back pain, weakness of the limbs, red tongue, taut pulse, onset caused by exasperation mean hyperactivity of the liver yang. Stuffiness in the chest, nausea, vomiting, poor appetite, mental restlessness, sticky yellow tongue coating, smooth pulse indicate interior retention of phlegm due to dampness.

Treatment

A. Body Acupuncture

a. Deficiency of qi and blood

Method: Activating the function of the Spleen and Kidney meridians is the key to treatment. The reinforcing method and/or moxibustion is used.

Prescription: Pishu (B 20), Shenshu (B 23), Guanyuan (CV 4), Zusanli (S 36).

Explanation: When vertigo is due to deficiency of qi and blood, treatment should aim at tonifying the spleen and kidney, therefore Pishu (B 20) and Shenshu (B 23) are chosen to strengthen the primary qi. Zusanli (S 36) is taken to promote transportation and transformation of food essence, facilitate production of qi and blood, and replenish the primary qi. Baihui (GV 20) and Guanyuan (CV 4) of the Governor Vessel and Conception Vessel meridians are used to strengthen qi and promote blood circulation. Sufficient qi and blood in the body may check vertigo.

b. Hyperactivity of the liver yang

Method: Points in the Liver and Gallbladder meridians are selected as the main points. Needling is done with the reinforcing method.

Prescription: Fengchi (G 20), Ganshu (B 18), Shenshu (B 23), Xingjian (Liv 2), Xiaxi (G 43).

Explanation: Fengchi (G 20) is used to dispel the upward floating yang. Xingjian (Liv 2) and Xiaxi (G 43) are chosen to reduce the floating weak yang of the liver and gallbladder. This is considered treatment for the secondary cause. Back-Shu points are used to regulate and tonify the liver and kidney, treating the root cause.

c. Interior retention of phlegm

Method: Treatment aims at regulating the middle burner and resolving phlegm. Needling is done with the reducing method.

Prescription: Zhongwan (CV 12), Neiguan (P 6), Fenglong (S 40), Jiexi (S 41).

Explanation: Zhongwan (CV 12) and Fenglong (S 40) are taken to remove the interior retention of phlegm. Neiguan (P 6) is prescribed for clearing fire from the heart and regulating the stomach qi, thus stopping vomiting. Jiexi (S 41) is used to lower the fire of the stomach and resolve phlegm indirectly, thus stopping vertigo.

B. Ear Acupuncture

Main points: Kidney, Ear Shenmen, Occiput, Inner Ear, Subcortex.

Method: Two or three points are used for each treatment. Needles are twirled intermittently with moderate or strong stimulation and retained for twenty to thirty minutes. Treatment is given once a day. Five to seven treatments make a course.

C. Scalp Acupuncture

Region for treatment: Dizziness and Auditory Region.

Method: Treatment is given once a day. Five to ten treatments make a course.

D. Point Injection

Main points: Hegu (LI 4), Taichong (Liv 3), Yiming (Extra 7) or Neiguan (P 6), Fengchi (G 20), Sidu (TE 9).

Method: Each point is injected with a 5 percent or 10 percent solution of 3 to 5 ml glucose or 0.5 ml vitamin B_{12}. Two or three points are used for each treatment. Treatment is given once every other day.

Remarks

The patient is advised to drink little water and eat lightly during an attack of auditory vertigo. If it is a vertiginous syndrome, the primary affection should be treated first.

22. Malaria

Malaria is a summer and autumn infectious disease caused by plasmodium infection. It is characterized by chills, high fever, sweating, etc.

Etiology and Pathology

Onset of malaria usually results from infection of pestilential factors accompanied by invasion of the semiexterior and semiinterior of the body by pathogenic wind, cold, summer heat and dampness. Relapse of prolonged malaria may result in consumption of qi and blood, retarded flow of qi by pathogenic dampness, phlegm formation due to concretion of body fluids and accumulation at the hypochondriac region. All are considered the source of malaria.

Differentiation

Malaria is marked by alternate chills and fevers, accompanied by sweating. It starts with lassitude and gooseflesh, followed by shaking chills, low back pain, consequent internal and external sensation of a burning body, splitting headache, flushed face and lips, extreme thirst. The fever subsides and the body feels cool after sweating. Tongue coating is white and sticky; pulse is taut and tense during attack of chills, rapid and smooth in fever. Malaria attacks periodically, so it may be classified as quotidian malaria, tertian malaria and quartan malaria. In prolonged cases lumps may appear in the left hypochondriac region with or without tenderness, which is called the source of malaria.

Treatment

A. Body Acupuncture

Method: Treatment aims at dispersing qi, dispelling the pathogenic factors and relieving the exterior symptoms. Needling is done with the reducing method. Treatment is given two to three hours before attack.

Prescription: Dazhui (GV 14), Houxi (SI 3), Jianshi (P 5).

Explanation: Dazhui (GV 14), the place where three yang meridians of the hand and foot intersect, is used to disperse and regulate the qi in the yang meridians, thus dispelling the pathogenic agents. Houxi (SI 3), the Jing (River) point of the Small Intestine Meridian of Hand-Taiyang, disperses the qi of the Taiyang and Governor Vessel meridians and eliminates the pestilential factors. Jianshi (P 5), pertaining to the Pericardium Meridian of Hand-Jueyin, is an empirical point in treatment of malaria. Selection of the three points can disperse the yang and dispel the pathogenic agents.

Modification: Prick Shixuan (Extra 30) if the tongue turns purple during attack. For cases with enlargement of the spleen, Zhangmen (Liv 13) and Pigen (Extra 20) should be added. For aperiodic attacks treatment is given twice daily. For cases with high fever one or two Jing (Well) points should be pricked until bleeding.

B. Ear Acupuncture

Main points: Adernal, Subcortex, Endocrine, Liver, Spleen.

Method: Needling is given one or two hours before the attack. Needles are retained for one hour. Three successive treatments make a course.

C. External Application Therapy

Method: A certain amount of fresh buttercup, wild peppermint or garlic is pounded into a paste. Neiguan (P 6) or Jianshi (P 5) is covered with the paste, fixed with adhesive plaster, for three to four hours. Treatment is given one or two hours before the attack.

Remarks

(1) Acupuncture treatment is more effective for tertian malaria. It is advisable to administer drugs for malignant malaria.

(2) It is usually thought that acupuncture treatment should be given two or three hours before the attack, but clinical observation indicates acupuncture is also effective during attack.

23. Jaundice

Jaundice is characterized by yellow sclera, skin and urine. The causative factors may be exogenous affection and internal injury, but pathological changes are usually in the liver, gallbladder, spleen and stomach. Conventional classifications and terms used for jaundice in traditional Chinese medicine are intricate, which makes for difficulty in differentiation. Here jaundice is grouped under yin and yang types by its nature.

Jaundice includes hepatogenic, obstructive and hemolytic types.

Etiology and Pathology

Jaundice is mainly caused by pathogenic dampness. In case of invasion of the body by pathogenic wind mixed with pathogenic dampness, after the wind has been dispelled, the retained dampness transforms into heat, lingering in the spleen and stomach. Then the liver and gallbladder are heated by the pathogenic dampness and heat, impeding the normal flow of bile, causing bile to penetrate the muscles and skin, thus causing jaundice. Irregular food intake and overstrain lead to weakness of the spleen and stomach and hypoactivity of yang of the middle burner. In this case pathogenic dampness transforms into cold. The retained cold and dampness also impede the normal flow of bile, causing bile to penetrate the muscles, skin and blood vessels, resulting in jaundice.

Differentiation

(1) Jaundice of yang type: Marked by bright yellow skin, fever, thirst, scant yellow urine, distension feeling in abdomen, constipation, stuffiness in chest, nausea, vomiting, sticky yellow tongue coating, smooth, rapid pulse.

(2) Jaundice of yin type: Manifested by dark yellow skin, lassitude, poor appetite, loose stool, aversion to cold, full feeling in the epigastrium and abdomen, pale tongue with sticky coating, deep, slow, weak pulse.

Treatment

A. Body Acupuncture

a. Jaundice of yang type

Method: Treatment aims at soothing the liver and gallbladder and promoting their function in excretion of bile to remove the dampness and heat. Needling is done with the reducing method.

Prescription: Danshu (B 19), Yanglingquan (G 34), Yinlingquan (Sp 9), Neiting (S 44), Taichong (Liv 3).

Explanation: Danshu (B 19) and Yanglingquan (G 34) are employed to eliminate the dampness and heat, as jaundice is usually caused by accumulation of damp heat in the gallbladder. Taichong (Liv 3) is used to smooth the flow of qi in the Liver and Gallbladder meridians. Yinlingquan (Sp 6), the He (Sea) point of the Foot-Taiyin Meridian, and Neiting (S 44), the Xing (Spring) point of the Foot-Yangming Meridian, are used in combination to drive the dampness and heat in the spleen and stomach downward to the urethra.

Modifications:

For cases with a full feeling in the epigastrium and poor appetite, Zhongwan (CV 12) and Zusanli (S 36) are added.

For cases with stuffiness in the chest, nausea and vomiting, Neiguan (P 6) and Gongsun (Sp 4) are added.

For cases with abdominal distension and constipation, Dachongshu (B 25) and Taianshu (S 25) are added.

b. Jaundice of yin type

Method: The principle of treatment is to strengthen the function of the spleen, promote secretion and excretion of bile, remove cold dampness by warming. Needling is done with the half reinforcing, half reducing method combined with moxibustion.

Prescription: Zhiyang (GV 9), Pishu (B 20), Danshu (B 19), Zhongwan (CV 12), Zusanli (S 36), Sanyinjiao (Sp 6).

Explanation: Strengthening and warming the spleen are taken as the key in treatment, since preponderance of cold dampness is the pathology of jaundice of yin type. Zhiyang (GV 9) is a point infused by the qi of the Governor Vessel Meridian. Needling and moxibustion are applied to warm and disperse the qi of the body. Zhongwan (CV 12), the influential point dominating the Fu organs, combined with Zusanli (S 36) and Pishu (B 20), is used with the reinforcing method to strengthen the function of the spleen and stomach, thus removing dampness. Danshu (B 19) is prescribed for facilitating the gallbladder to secrete and excrete bile. Sanyinjiao (Sp 6) is taken to conduct the pathogenic dampness downwards.

Modifications:

For cases with aversion to cold, Mingmen (GV 4) and Qihai (CV 6) are added.

For cases with loose stool, Tianshu (S 25) and Guanyuan (CV 4) are added.

Remarks

Acupuncture treatment is more effective for hepatogenic jaundice. Sterilization and isolation should be strictly administered during the acute stage. Jaundice caused by other factors should be treated by herbs or a combination of Chinese and Western medicine. Acupuncture treatment is a secondary measure.

24. Edema

Edema in traditional Chinese medicine is also known as hydropic disease and puffiness, which generally refers to puffiness of the head, face, eyelids, four limbs, abdomen and back, or a general dropsy. The cause is believed to be dysfunction of the triple burners in qi transformation. The lung, spleen and kidney are involved in pathological changes. Edema as described in ancient Chinese medical literature includes acute and chronic nephritis, congestive cardiac failure, cirrhosis and malnutrition.

Etiology and Pathology

Normal circulation and distribution of body fluids depend on proper functioning of the lung qi in regulating water passage, of the spleen in transportation and transformation, and of the kidney in control of water retention and excretion. The triple burners dominate water passage, enabling the urinary bladder to function normally and urination to be unobstructed. In case of dysfunction of the triple burners obstruction of qi flow and retention of fluid exudate occur. When the abnormal excretion of metabolized water permeates the skin and muscles, edema results. If the edema is due to invasion by exogenous pathogenic wind, leading to failure of the lung qi to disperse, inability of the lung to regulate water passage and retention and overflow of water, it is considered a yang type. If overstrain and uncontrolled sexual activities injure the spleen and kidney, causing inability of the yang of the spleen and kidney to vaporize body fluids, it is usually believed a yin type.

Differentiation

(1) Yang type: Onset is usually abrupt. Mild edema first appears on the face and

eyelids, followed by a general edema, lustrous skin, swelling of the scrotum, stuffiness in the chest, shortness of breath, scant yellow urine, superficial, smooth pulse, sticky white tongue coating.

(2) Yin type: Onset is usually insidious. Initial symptom is mild edema on the dorsum of the foot. Later on puffiness gradually covers the whole body. Accompanying symptoms are pallor, clear urine or scant loose stool, aversion to cold, deep and thin or slow pulse.

Treatment

Principle of treatment is to regulate the passage of qi of the triple burners. For yang syndrome the lung and kidney should be concerned. Needling is done with the reducing method. Moxibustion is not advisable in general. Yin syndrome should be treated by strengthening the function of the spleen and kidney with the reinforcing method. Moxibustion is usually applied.

Prescription: Shuifen (CV 9), Qihai (CV 6), Sanyinjiao (Sp 6), Zusanli (S 36), Sanjiaoshu (B 22).

Yang syndrome: Feishu (B 15), Dazhu (B 11), Hegu (LI 4).

Yin syndrome: Pishu (B 20), Shenshu (B 23).

Explanation: This prescription is mainly to strengthen water metabolism, for which Sanjiaoshu (B 22) is used. Qihai (CV 6) is selected to activate the qi. Shuifen (CV 9), pertaining to the Governor Vessel Meridian located at the small intestine, is taken to distinguish part of the refined materials of water and grain. Thus it is a key point in treating retention of metabolized water. Zusanli (S 36) and Sanyinjiao (B 22) regulate the qi of the Foot Taiyin and Yangming meridians and promote the smooth functioning of the spleen and stomach in order to restore normal dispersion and distribution of body fluids. For yang syndrome, pertaining to the exterior, Feishu (B 13) and Dazhu (B 11) are prescribed to disperse the qi in the lung and the Foot-Taiyang Meridian. The Hand-Yangming Meridian is externally and internally related with the Hand-Taiyin Meridian, therefore Hegu (LI 4) is used to help the lung in regulating water metabolism and conducting downward flow water to the urinary bladder. Yin syndrome is due to exhaustion of the kidney yang and deficiency in the spleen, resulting in disturbance of water metabolism and hyperactivity of yang in the stomach and spleen. Shenshu (B 23) is selected to warm the kidney yang and Pishu (B 20) is used to strengthen the transporting and transforming functions of the spleen, thus removing pathogenic water.

Modifications:

For cases with swelling of the face, Shuigou (GV 26) is added.

For cases with swelling of the upper limbs, Pianli (LI 16) is added.

For cases with swelling of the lower limbs, Yinlingquan (Sp 9) is added.

Remarks

(1) The primary cause of edema should be investigated. Meanwhile, both herbs and Western drugs may be administered.

(2) Patients are advised to take bed rest, keep warm and prevent common colds. Avoid salty food and drink fewer beverages. When edema is relieved, patients are allowed to have low-salt food.

25. Testis Pain and Swelling

The onset of disorders marked by testis pain and/or swelling is often related to troubles in the Conception Vessel and Liver meridians of Foot-Jueyin.

Etiology and Pathology

Testis pain and swelling due to cold are caused by stagnation of qi and blood in the Conception Vessel and Liver meridians due to exposure to cold, dampness and wind.

Testis pain and swelling due to dampness and heat are caused by affection of the Conception Vessel and Foot-Jueyin meridians due to downward invasion of dampness and heat.

Noticeable or unnoticeable testis pain and swelling are caused by qi deficiency and stinking of qi due to overstrain.

Differentiation

Testis disorder is manifested by lower abdominal pain, radiating the testis, and swelling and distending pain of the testis and scrotum.

(1) Testis pain and swelling due to cold are characterized by pain in the scrotum with a cold sensation, heaviness, contraction of the testis, causing lateral lower abdominal pain, thin white tongue coating, deep, thin pulse.

(2) Testis pain and swelling due to dampness and heat are manifested by swelling of the scorme with a hot sensation, distension pain in the testis, chills and fever, yellow urine, constipation, yellow coated tongue, taut, rapid pulse.

(3) Noticeable or unnoticeable testis pain and swelling: Symptoms are synesthesialgia and distending pain in the groin and scrotum. A part of the small intestine descends into the scrotum when the patient stands up and disappears when the patient lies flat. Enlargement of the scrotum occurs in a prolonged case.

Treatment

(1) Testis pain and swelling due to cold

Method: Main points are in the Conception Vessel and Liver meridians of Foot-Jueyin. The reducing method is used. Moxibustion may also be applied.

Prescription: Guanyuan (CV 4), Sanyinjiao (Sp 6), Dadun (Liv 1).

Explanation: It is caused by disorders of Conception Vessel Meridian. The Foot-Jueyin Meridian curves around the external genitalia. The three yin foot meridians intersect at the Governor Vessel Meridian. Therefore, Guanyuan (CV 4) of the Conception Vessel Meridian, Dadun (Liv 3) of the Liver Meridian and Sanyinjiao (Sp 6), a crossing point of the three yin foot meridians, are selected to remove obstructions in the meridians. Moxibustion applied to them warms the meridian and dispel cold, further relieving the acute lower abdominal pain.

(2) Testis pain and swelling due to dampness and heat

Method: Main points are in the Conception Vessel, Foot-Jueyin and Taiyin meridians. Needling is given with the reducing method.

Prescription: Guanyuan (CV 4), Guilai (S 29), Taichong (Liv 3), Yinlingquan (Sp 9), Sanyinjiao (Sp 6).

Explanation: Guanyuan (CV 4) and Taichong (Liv 3) are taken to expel accumulated heat in the Foot-Jueyin and the Conception Vessel meridians. Because the Foot-Yangming Meridian meets the external genitalia at the anterior privates, Guilai (S 29) is used as a supplementary point. Yinlingquan (Sp 9) and Sanyinjiao (Sp 6) are prescribed for driving the dampness and heat away from the water passage. As a result, swelling and pain with a hot sensation of the scrotum will be relieved gradually.

(3) Noticeable or unnoticeable testis pain and swelling

Method: Points in the Conception Vessel Meridian are mainly selected. Moxibustion is applied.

Prescription: Guanyuan (CV 4), Sanguojiu (Extra), Dadun (Liv 1)

Explanation: Guanyuan (CV 4), believed to be the outlet of qi in the triple burners, is chosen to strengthen its function in holding and keeping the internal organs in position. Moxibustion applied to Sanguojiu (Extra) can help Guanyuan (CV 4) to raise the sunken qi. Dadun (Liv 1), pertaining to the Liver Meridian of Foot-Jueyin and curving around the external genitalia, is a very important point in treatment of testis pain and swelling.

Remarks

Acupuncture treatment can relieve symptoms. For severe cases with frequent attacks surgical operation should be taken into consideration.

26. Beriberi

Beriberi is characterized by weakness of the lower limbs and difficulty in walking, therefore it is also known as asthenic foot in traditional Chinese medicine. As clinical manifestations vary, beriberi includes two types, dry and wet.

Etiology and Pathology

Beriberi is caused by invasion of the lower limbs by pathogenic dampness and cold and dampness and heat, which permeate the skin, muscles and tendons, or by irregular food intake, resulting in impairment of the spleen and stomach and downward infusion of pathogenic dampness and heat. Sometimes it is due to hypofunction of the spleen and long-standing dampness and heat, leading to deficiency of qi and blood and malnourishment of the tendons and vessels.

Differentiation

The onset is manifested only by weakness of the foot, followed gradually by a feeling of heaviness, intractable numbness, or puffiness. Clinically there are two types, dry and wet.

(1) The wet type pertains to the excess syndrome, marked by puffiness of the dorsum of the foot or the whole leg, slow pulse, and sticky white tongue coating.

(2) The dry type pertains to the deficiency syndrome manifested by gradual emaciation of the calf and shin, intractable numbness, a feeling of haviness or sometimes constipation, yellow urine, light-red tongue, taut, rapid pulse. In prolonged cases shortness of breath due to upward perversive flow of qi, palpitation, fever with irritability, vomiting, loss of appetite, semiconsciousness, considered a critical condition called "beriberi raiding the heart," appear.

Treatment

A. Body Acupuncture

Method: Main points are in the Foot-Shaoyang, Yangming and Taiyin meridians. The reducing method is used for the wet type. Moxibustion is advisable for cases with abundant cold. The dry type is treated by the reinforcing or half reinforcing, half reducing method. For cases with abundant heat, moxibustion is not advisable.

Prescription: Yanglingquan (G 34), Zusanli (S 36), Xuanzhong (G 39), Sanyinjiao (Sp 6).

Deficiency in the spleen and stomach: Pishu (B 20) and Weishu (B 20).

Explanation: Invasion of the body by pathogenic dampness, starting in the lower limbs, first results in retention of dampness in the skin, muscles and tendons. Zusanli (S 36) and Sanyinjiao (Sp 6) are chosen to eliminate dampness in the Yangming and Taiyin meridians. Yanglingquan (G 34), Xuanzhong (G 39), two of the eight influential points, activate the qi flow and strengthen tendons and bones.

Modification: For cases of "beriberi raiding the heart" Guanyuan (CV 4), Jueque (CV 14) and Neiguan (P 6) are added.

B. Electroacupuncture

Main points: Fengshi (C 31), Zusanli (S 36), Femur-Futu (S 32), Xuanzhong (G 39).

Method: Electric stimulation is applied for ten to fifteen minutes. Stimulating capacity and frequency of the electric pulse are adjusted according to the tolerance of patients.

Remarks

(1) Acupuncture treatment integrated with herbs and Western drugs and massage can improve curative effects. "Beriberi raiding the heart" must be given timely treatment by combining traditional and Western medicine, as it is an acute, critical case.

(2) It is advisable for patients to eat more red beans, Job's-tears seeds, peanuts and Chinese dates to regulate and strengthen the function of the spleen and stomach.

27. Headache

Headache is a subjective symptom, usually seen in various kinds of acute and chronic diseases. Here we shall discuss only headache related to obstruction of collaterals by stagnant blood, hyperactivity of the liver yang, and deficiency of qi and blood. Headache as a secondary symptom of other disorders will not be discussed here.

Headache is usually seen in hypertension, intracavitary tumour, neurosis, migraine, infectious and febrile diseases.

Etiology and Pathology

Headache occurs because of upward invasion of the collaterals by pathogenic wind and cold. It leads to disharmony of qi and blood, obstruction of the meridians and collaterals, and long-standing stagnation of blood in the meridians, caused by a sudden weather change or occasional exposure to the wind. Dysfunction of the liver results in depression, qi later turning into fire to disturb the mind. This is another cause of headache. Agitation and upward disturbance of wind of the liver and gallbladder along their course of the meridians can also cause headache. In cases of congenital weakness, constant deficiency of qi and blood, insufficiency of the reservoir of medulla or mental strain may also cause headache.

Differentiation

(1) Invasion of the meridians and collaterals by pathogenic wind is characterized by paroxysmal attacks with stabbing and stationary pain. In severe cases swelling appears on the scalp. Generally there are no accompanying symptoms. This type is also called head wind.

(2) Hyperactivity of the liver yang is marked by headache with vertigo, pain appearing on either side of the head, mental restlessness, irritability, flushed face, bitter taste in the mouth, taut, rapid pulse, red tongue with yellow coating.

(3) Deficiency of qi and blood is manifested by an insidious headache with dizziness and heaviness, blurring of vision, lassitude, pallor, aversion to cold, headache intensified by mental strain, thin, weak pulse, thin white tongue coating.

Treatment

A. Body Acupuncture

a. Invasion of the meridians and collaterals by pathogenic wind

Method: Select points located on the head. Needling is done with the reducing method and needles are retained for some minutes. The affected area is tapped heavily with plum-blossom needles until slight bleeding occurs.

Prescriptions:

Vertical headache: Baihui (GV 20), Tongtian (B 7), Xingjian (Liv 2), Ahshi points.

Frontal headache: Shangxing (GV 23), Touwei (S 38), Hegu (LI 4), Ahshi points.

Occipital headache: Houding (GV 19), Tianzhu (B 10), Kunlun (B 60), Ahshi points.

Explanation: As persistent headache affects meridians, plum-blossom needling is applied to cause bleeding. This is known as "a method for removing depression and stagnation." A relapse headache due to pathogenic wind may be treated in this way. The above points are prescribed depending on the course of the meridians, and points on the affected and distal areas are combined to remove obstructions in the meridians.

b. Hyperactive yang of the liver

Method: Main points are in the Foot-Jueyin and Shaoyang meridians. The reducing method is applied.

Prescription: Fengchi (G 20), Baihui (GV 20), Xuanlu (G 5), Xiaxi (G 43), Xingjian (Liv 2).

Explanation: The Liver Meridian of Foot-Jueyin meets the Governor Vessel Meridian at the vertex. The Gallbladder Meridian of Foot-Shaoyang runs on both sides of the head. Points on the affected area of these two meridians and distal points are used in combination with the reducing method to eliminate heat and check the hyperfunctioning of wind.

c. Deficiency of qi and blood

Method: Main points are in the Governor Vessel Meridian and the Back-Shu points. Needling is done with the reinforcing method. Moxibustion may also be applied.

Prescription: Baihui (GV 20), Qihai (CV 6), Ganshu (B 18), Pishu (B 20), Shenshu

(B 23), Hegu (LI 4), Zusanli (S 36).

Explanation: The Back-Shu points of the liver, spleen and kidney are selected because the liver stores blood, the spleen unites blood and the brain's reservoir of medulla originates in the kidney. Puncturing Qihai (CV 6) can promote growth of the primary qi. Baihui (GV 20) is chosen to invigorate the vital function. Hegu (LI 4) and Zusanli (S 36) regulate the qi in the Yangming meridians. This is believed to be a treatment for the root cause.

B. Moxibustion with Warming Needle

Thicker filiform needles are used to puncture Fengfu (GV 16) and Yamen (GV 15) with the ignited moxa cone fixed on the handle of the needle. One or two points are taken with three to five moxa cones burned for each treatment. Treatment is given once a day or every other day for headache due to deficiency and cold.

C. Cutaneous Needling

Taiyang (Extra 2), Yintang (Extra 1) and Ahshi points are tapped heavily until bleeding, followed by cupping, for headache due to invasion of the meridians by pathogenic wind and hyperactivity of the liver yang.

D. Ear Acupuncture

Main points: Occiput, Forehead, Subcortex, Ear Shenmen.

Method: Two or three points are needled for each treatment. Needles are retained for twenty to thirty minutes and twirled every five minutes, or intradermal needles are embedded in the points for three to seven days. Prick the retroauricular veins with a three-edged needle to cause bleeding for persistent headache.

E. Point Injection

Find the sensitive spots at the medial and superior angle of the scapular close to Tianliao (TE 15) and then quickly inject 15 ml of 10 percent glucose into the selected points on the upper part of the scapular spine. A distending pain occurs. Treatment is given once every other day or every two days for migraine. In treatment of persistent headache a mixture of 3.5 ml of 0.25 percent procaine and 0.5 ml caffeine is prepared; 0.5 to 1 ml is for each point, or 0.1 ml of the mixture is injected into the tender sports.

Remarks

If headache does not respond to acupuncture treatment or becomes worse, introcranial disorders should be taken into consideration. Treat primary affection first.

28. Hypochondariac Pain

Hypochondriac pain refers to pain in one or both sides of the hypochondriac region. It is a subjective symptom frequently seen clinically. It is pointed out in the "Treatise on the Five Pathogenic Agents, Miraculous Pivot," that "pathogenic agents staying in the liver lead to hypochondriac pain." The Liver Meridian runs through the hypochondriac region and the liver is united with the gallbladder in a functional yoke. This shows that hypochondriac pain is closely related to the liver and gallbladder.

Hypochondriac pain may be seen in acute or chronic disorders of the liver, gallbladder, pleurae and so on.

Etiology and Pathology

The liver is situated in the hypochondriac region, but its meridians spread to both upper sides of the body. Emotional depression leads to dysfunction of the liver and obstruction of its collaterals. Then stagnation of qi results in hypochondriac pain. Another cause of hypochondriac pain is depletion of essence and blood and malnourishment of the Liver Meridian, or qi and blood stagnation of the collaterals caused by contusion and sprain.

Differentiation

Hypochondriac pain often occurs on one costal side, in some cases on both sides. If it is due to exasperation and emotional depression, symptoms are distending pain in the costal and hypochondriac region, fullness in the chest, poor appetite, taut pulse. This is known as depression of the liver qi. If it is caused by contusion and sprain, there is sharp stabbing and fixed pain. This is believed to be stagnation of qi and blood. The above two disorders contribute to an excess syndrome. Hypochondriac pain due to deficiency of essence and blood is believed to be a deficiency syndrome, marked by insidious hypochondriac pain, red tongue with little coating, thin, rapid pulse.

Treatment

A. Body Acupuncture

a. Excess syndrome

Method: Main points are in the Foot-Jueyin and Shaoyang meridians. Needling is given with the reducing method.

Prescription: Qimen (Liv 14), Zhigou (TE 6), Yanglingquan (G 34), Zusanli (S 36), Taichong (Liv 3).

Explanation: The liver is united with the gallbladder in their functional yoke. Their meridians spread over the hypochondriac regions. Hence, Qimen (Liv 14) and Taichong (Liv 3), combined with Zhigou (TE 6) and Yanglingquan (G 34), are used to invigorate the flow of qi in the liver and gallbladder and to kill pain. Zusanli (S 36) harmonizes and lowers the stomach qi and removes fullness from the hypochondriac region.

b. Deficiency syndrome

Method: The Back-Shu points and those in the Foot-Jueyin Meridian are chiefly prescribed. Needling is done with the reinforcing or half reinforcing half reducing method.

Prescription: Ganshu (B 18), Shenshu (B 23), Qimen (Liv 14), Xingjian (Liv 2), Zusanli (S 36), Sanyinjiao (Sp 6).

Explanation: Ganshu (B 18) and Shenshu (B 23) are punctured with the reinforcing method to replenish the yin of the liver and kidney. Qimen (Liv 14), the Front-Mu point of the liver, is taken as a local point to regulate the liver qi. Xingjian (Liv 2) is chosen to eliminate the heat due to deficiency in the meridians. Zusanli (S 36) and Sanyinjiao (Sp 6) are cooperatively used to strengthen the function of the spleen and stomach, the source of transformation of the human body.

B. Cutaneous Needling

Cutaneous needling applied to the chest and hypochondriac region first, then associated with cupping, is most helpful for hypochondriac pain due to overstrain.

C. Point Injection

Inject 10 ml of 10 percent glucose, or add 1 ml vitamin B_{12} into the Huatuo Jiaji points. The syringe needle should be inserted into the area near the affected root of the intercostal nerve. When the needling is clearly felt, lift the syringe needle a little, then inject the solution. Several points are used for each treatment. The treatment is for costal neuralgia.

D. Ear Acupuncture

Main points: Chest, Ear Shenmen, Liver.

Method: Two or three points on the involved side are taken. Needles are retained for twenty to thirty minutes. Treatment is given during the attack.

Remarks

Clinical examinations should be done during acupuncture treatment. When necessary, morbid factors must be removed first.

29. Epigastric Pain

Stomachache in traditional Chinese medicine refers to pain in the epigastric region. It is a common and recurrent syndrome. As the pain is near the xyphoid region, it is also called cardiac and abdominal pain and cardiac pain but it is different from "true heart pain" described in the *Inner Classic of the Yellow Sovereign.* This syndrome is frequently seen in gastritis, gastric ulcer, gastroneurosis, and so on.

Etiology and Pathology

The stomach is united with the spleen in their functional yoke, and the free movement of the liver qi can promote the function of the spleen and stomach in transportation. That is why stomachache is closely related to the liver and spleen. Causative factors are described as follows:

(1) Invasion of the stomach by the liver qi: Melancholy, anxiety, exasperation and mental depression injure the liver, resulting in dysfunction of the liver in maintaining the free flow of qi. When rebel liver qi attacks the stomach and retards the passage of qi, epigastric pain occurs.

(2) Weakness and cold of the spleen and stomach: Congenital insufficiency or constant deficiency in the middle burner leads to breeding of interior cold. As a result, epigastric pain is usually induced easily by irregular food intake, anxiety, overstrain or exposure to cold.

Differentiation

(1) Invasion of the stomach by the liver qi is marked by fullness and distending sensation in the epigastrium, pain radiating to the hypochondriac region, frequent belching or regurgitation of sour and bitter fluid, thick white tongue coating, deep, taut pulse.

(2) Weakness and cold of the spleen and stomach are manifested by insidious pain in the epigastrium, regurgitation of thin fluid, aversion to cold, pain relieved by pressure, lassitude, white tongue coating, weak, soft pulse.

Treatment

A. Body Acupuncture

a. Invasion of the stomach by the liver qi

Method: Main points are in the Foot-Jueyin and Yangming meridians. Needling is done with the reducing method.

Prescription: Zhongwan (CV 12), Qimen (Liv 14), Neiguan (P 6), Zusanli (S 36), Yanglingquan (G 34).

Explanation: Zhongwan (CV 12) and Zusanli (S 36) are used to regulate the stomach qi in descending and ascending. Neiguan (P 6) is prescribed for relieving depression. Qimen (Liv 14) and Yanglingquan (G 34) are taken to check the rebel qi of the liver and gallbladder, enabling the liver qi to be pacified and the stomach qi to descend.

b. Weakness and cold of the spleen and stomach

Method: The Back-Shu points and those in the Conception Vessel Meridian are mainly selected. Needling is done with the reinforcing method. Moxibustion may be used in combination.

Prescription: Pishu (B 20), Weishu (B 21), Zhongwan (CV 12), Zhangmen (Liv 13), Neiguan (P 6), Zusanli (S 36).

Explanation: As weakness and cold of the spleen and stomach are due to yang deficiency of the middle burner, Back-Shu points and Front-Mu points, such as Weishu (B 21), Zhongwan (CV 12), Pishu (B 20) and Zhangmen (Liv 13), are mainly used in combination to invigorate the yang of the middle burner. Points below the knee and elbow, such as Neiguan (P 6) and Zusanli (S 36), are used in coordination to regulate the stomach qi and check pain.

B. Cupping

Points of the upper abdomen and back are selected for cupping after acupuncture treatment for epigastric pain due to weakness and cold.

C. Ear Acupuncture

Main points: Stomach, Spleen, Sympathetic Nerve, Ear Shenmen, Subcortex.

Method: Select three to five points for each treatment. Needles are retained for thirty minutes. Sometimes electroacupuncture or needle embedding is used. For cases with epigastric pain and acidity, Endocrine is selected instead of Stomach. For cases of duodenal ulcer, Duodenum should be added.

D. Point-embedding Therapy

Main points:

Group 1: Zusanli (S 36) on the left, Weishu (B 21) towards Pishu (B 20).

Group 2: Zhongwan (CV 12) towards Shangwan (CV 13), Zusanli (S 36) on the right.

Group 3: Xiawan (CV 10), Lintai (GV 10), Liangmen (S 21).

Method: The three groups of points are taken alternately. Treatment is given every twenty to thirty days.

E. Point Injection

Main points: Weishu (B 21), Pishu (B 20), Huatuo Jiaji points corresponding to their own zang-fu organs, Zhongwan (CV 12), Neiguan (P 6), Zusanli (S 36).

Method: One to three points are injected with a dosage of solution of saffron, Chinese angelica, atropine or procaine. Dosage is determined by the individual condition.

Remarks

(1) Sometimes epigastric pain and disorder of the gallbladder, liver, and pancreas are very much alike, so correct diagnosis is important.

(2) Ulcerative bleeding and perforation of the stomach due to ulcer are critical conditions that should be treated promptly by surgery or other measures.

(3) Regular meals are advised. Pungent foods should be avoided.

30. Abdominal Pain

Abdominal pain often accompanies various disorders of the visceral organs. Abdominal pain caused by dysentery, stomachache, hernia, intestinal carbuncle and disorders such as those connected with menstruation will not be discussed in this section. Causative factors other than the above are mentioned here.

Etiology and Pathology

(1) Interior accumulation of cold due to frequent intake of too much raw and cold food and interior breeding of cold in the body or to invasion of the abdominal region by pathogenic wind and cold results in abdominal pain.

(2) Constant deficiency of yang in the spleen, causing dysfunction in transportation and transformation, allows the easy inducement of abdominal pain by any invasion of cold, overeating or hunger and overstrain.

(3) Retention of food due to overeating of greasy and pungent food leads to dysfunction of the stomach and intestines in digestion and transmission and obstruction of the qi passage.

Differentiation

(1) Interior accumulation of cold is marked by a sudden, violent abdominal pain that responds to warmth and is aggravated by cold, loose stool, cold limbs, pale tongue with moist white coating, deep, tense pulse.

(2) Deficiency of yang in the spleen is marked by insidious pain alleviated by pressure, loose stool, lassitude, aversion to cold, thin white tongue coating, deep, thin pulse.

(3) Retention of food is manifested by fullness of the epigastric region and abdomen, pain aggravated by pressure, anorexia, foul belching, sour regurgitation or abdominal pain accompanied by a strong desire to have a bowel movement, after which the pain is alleviated, sticky tongue coating, smooth pulse.

Treatment

A. Body Acupuncture

a. Interior accumulation of cold

Method: Main points are in the Foot-Taiyin and Yangming meridians. Needling is done with the reducing method. Indirect moxibustion with salt to Shenque (CV 8) is prescribed.

Prescription: Zhongwan (CV 12), Shenque (CV 8), Guanyuan (CV 4), Zusanli (S 36), Gongsun (Sp 4).

Explanation: Zhongwan (CV 12) is chosen to send the essence upward and the waste downward, regulating the qi in the stomach and intestine. To strengthen the function of the spleen and stomach. Zusanli (S 36) and Gongsun (Sp 4) are employed. Moxibustion to Shenque (CV 8) and Guanyuan (CV 4) warms the lower burner to remove a accumulated cold.

b. Deficiency of yang in the spleen

Method: Back-Shu points and points in the Conception Vessel Meridian are chiefly selected. Needling is done with the reinforcing method and moxibustion is applied.

Prescription: Pishu (B 20), Weishu (B 21), Zhongwan (CV 12), Zusanli (S 36), Qihai (CV 6), Zhangmen (Liv 13).

Explanation: Pishu (B 20), Weishu (B 21), Zhongwan (CV 12), one of the eight influential points, Zhangmen (Liv 13), one of the Front-Mu points, are prescribed for activating the yang in the spleen and stomach. Qihai (CV 6) and Zusanli (S 36) are selected to promote the transporting and digesting functions of the spleen and stomach.

c. Retention of food

Method: Points in the Conception Vessel and Foot-Yangming meridians are chiefly selected. Needling is done with the reducing method. Moxibustion is used in combination.

Prescription: Zhongwan (CV 12), Tianshu (S 25), Qihai (CV 6), Zusanli (S 36), sole Neiting (Extra).

Explanation: Zhongwan (CV 12), Zusanli (S 36), Tianshu (S 25) and Qihai (CV 6) are used to adjust the function of the stomach and intestines. Sole Neiting (Extra), an empirical point, is taken to eliminate retention of food. The above points used in combination enable the spleen, stomach and intestines to work smoothly.

B. Ear Acupuncture

Main points: Sympathetic Nerve, Ear Shenmen, Subcortex, Stomach, Spleen, Small Intestine.

Method: Three to five points are punctured with moderate stimulation. Needles are retained for ten to thirty minutes. Treatment is given once a day.

Remarks

Acupuncture treatment is quite effective for abdominal pain. For cases of abdominal pain due to acute abdominal disease, patients should be observed carefully. When necessary, medical consultation should take place in order to take appropriate and timely measures.

31. Low Back Pain

Low back pain is also known as pain in the lumbur region and spine. It is a common complaint. The lumbar is closely related to the kidney and connected with meridians in the back, so the kidney contributes to low back pain. Low back pain frequently occurs in sprain of the soft tissues in the lumbar region and muscular rheumatism or disorders of the spine and internal organs. Here, only low back pain due to damp cold, lumbar muscular strain and deficiency in the kidney is discussed.

Etiology and Pathology

Low back pain due to dampness and cold usually occurs after exposure to pathogenic wind-cold and dampness, which stay in the meridians and cause obstruction. Lumbar muscle strain is another cause of low back pain. An incomplete recovery after contusion and sprain or traumatic injury leads to deprivation of qi and blood, blood stasis and functional disturbances of the meridians. Low back pain due to deficiency in the kidney is caused by sexual indulgence, impairing the kidney and leading to deprivation of the kidney essense.

Differentiation

Low back pain due to dampness and cold usually occurs after invasion of pathogenic wind, cold and dampness. Symptoms are stiffness of the muscles, pain and a heavy sensation, the pain radiating to the spine, buttocks and lower limbs. If it is a prolonged case, relapse is caused by sudden weather changes. The pain worsens on cold, wet days. Low back pain due to strain often refers to strain in the lumbar region, which is intensified by overwork. There may be stiffness in this area. The pain is fixed and aggravated by turning the lumbar.

Low back pain due to deficiency in the kidney has the following symptoms: Insidious onset, mild and protracted pain, weakness of the lumbar region. If it is accompanied by lassitude, cold limbs, involuntary emission, and thin pulse, it shows yang deficiency in the kidney. If there is restlessness, yellow urine, rapid pulse, and red tongue, the pain is caused by yin deficiency in the kidney.

Treatment

Method: Main points are in the Foot-Taiyang and Governor Vessel meridians. The reinforcing, reducing or half reinforcing, half reducing method and/or moxibustion is used depending on the individual case.

Prescription: Shenshu (B 23), Weizhong (B 40), local Shu points or Ahshi points. Dampness and cold type: Fengfu (GV 16), Yaoyangguan (GV 3).

Lumbar muscle strain: Geshu (B 17), Ciliao (B 30).

Deficiency in the kidney: Mingmen (GV 4), Zhishi (B 52), Taixi (K 3).

Explanation: The kidney is located in the lumbar region, hence Shenshu (B 23) is selected to regulate the function of the kidney. Moxibustion can eliminate dampness and cold in the lumbar region. The meridian of the urinary bladder runs along both sides of the spine, reaches the lumbar and connects the kidney. Weizhong (B 40) as a distal point, therefore, is selected according to the course of its meridian to regulate the meridian qi of the urinary bladder. Points in the affected area or Ahshi points are taken as local points. Fengfu (GV 16) and Yaoyangguan (GV 3) are points in the Governor Vessel Meridian. The former eliminates wind and cold, while the two in combination disperse the yang qi. Geshu (B 17), the influential point, dominates blood. Weizhong (B 40), the Xi (Cleft) point, and Ciliao (B 32) enable the qi of the Urinary-Bladder Meridian to circulate freely and remove obstruction. They are most helpful for pain due to lumbar muscle strain. Application of moxibustion to Mingmen (GV 4) and needling Zhishi (B 52) with the reinforcing method can invigorate the yang in the kidney. Taixi (K 3), the

Yuan (Source) point of Foot-Shaoyin Meridian, is prescribed on the principle of the source point of the zang organ being selected to treat that organ.

Modification: In severe attack Weizhong (B 40) is pricked with a three-edged needle until bleeding. Generally, cupping may be applied too.

Remarks

Acupuncture treatment can obtain good results in treating various kinds of low back pain. If it is due to a vertebral tumour, it is not advisable to give acupuncture treatment to the involved area. The primary affection should be treated first.

32. Obstruction Syndromes

Obstruction syndromes are due to invasion of the meridians by pathogenic agents, resulting in retardation of qi and blood and leading to their impeded circulation, causing pain, numbness, a heavy sensation in the limbs and joints, and stiff muscles.

The disorders may include rheumatic fever, rheumatic arthritis, rheumatoid arthritis, and fibrositis.

Etiology and Pathology

There are many causative factors for the syndromes. They usually result from weakness of the defensive qi, overstrain and exposure to wind after sweating or cold in water and dampness. The pathogenic wind, cold and dampness invade the interior and obstruct the meridians. It is stated in the "Treatise on Obstruction Syndromes" of the *Inner Classic of the Yellow Sovereign* that "attack of wind, cold and dampness causes obstruction syndromes." In addition, if one usually has excessive heat in the interior of the body and is affected by pathogenic wind, cold and dampness, obstruction syndromes with fever will result when the pathogenic factors turn to heat.

Differentiation

(1) Obstruction syndromes due to dampness and wind: Main manifestations are arthralgia, numbness and heaviness of certain muscles in prolonged cases, contraction of the limbs due to swelling of joints. The syndromes are also divided into the following three types in view of their causes:

a. Wandering obstruction syndrome is marked by wandering pain in the joints of the limbs, chills and fever, sticky yellow tongue coating, shallow pulse.

b. Painful obstruction syndrome: General or local fixed joint pain alleviated by warmth and aggravated by cold, white coated tongue, taut, tense pulse.

c. Fixed obstruction syndrome is manifested by numbness of the muscles, fixed joint pain of the limbs with attacks provoked by cold wet weather and wind, sticky white tongue coating, weak, slow pulse.

(2) Obstruction syndromes with fever: Syndromes are joint pain, tenderness, motion impairment, fever, thirst, dry, yellow tongue coating, smooth, rapid pulse.

Treatment

A. Body Acupuncture

Method: Local points in the involved area and distal points on the course of the affected meridians are mainly prescribed. Ahshi points may also be chosen. Wandering and febrile obstruction syndromes are treated by puncturing superficially; the reducing method and plum-blossom needling may also be applied. For painful obstruction syndrome, moxibustion is often applied. Needles are inserted deep and retained. For cases with severe pain, the intradermal needle of thumbtack type or indirect moxibustion with ginger may also be administered. The fixed pain obstruction syndrome is treated by acupuncture and moxibustion or warm needling, plum-blossom needling and cupping.

Prescriptions:

Selection of the local points in individual cases:

Shoulder region: Jianyu (LI 15), Jianliao (TE 14), Naoshu (SI 10).

Elbow and upper arm: Quchi (LI 11), Hegu (LI 4), Tianjing (TE 10), Waiguan (TE 5), Chize (L 5).

Wrist region: Yangchi (TE 4), Waiguan (TE 5), Yangxi (LI 5), Hand Wangu (SI 4).

Vertebra: Shuigou (GV 26), Shenzhu (GV 12), Yaoyangguan (GV 3).

Hip region: Huantiao (G 30), Femur Juliao (G 29), Xuanzhong (G 39).

Femoral region: Zhibian (B 54), Chenfu (B 36), Yanglingquan (G 34).

Knee joints: Dubi (S 35), Liangqiu (S 34), Yanglingquan (G 34), Xiyangguan (G 33).

Ankle: Shenmai (B 62), Zhaohai (K 6), Kunlun (UB 60), Qiuxu (G 40).

Modifications:

For wandering syndrome, Geshu (B 17) and Xuehai (Sp 10) are added.

For painful syndrome, Shenshu (B 23) and Guanyuan (CV 4) are added.

For fixed pain, Zusanli (S 36) and Shangqiu (Sp 5) are added.

For obstruction syndrome with fever, Quchi (LI 11) is added.

Explanation: The above prescribed points are based on the running course of the involved channels. The purpose is to promote circulation of qi and blood and remove wind, cold and dampness from the channels. When obstruction is gone, the pain will be relieved subsequently. If the skin and muscles are involved, puncture superficially and use points in the affected area. If the tendons and bones are involved, deep needling is applied to the points with retention of needles. Various treatments and manipulations are employed for different cases. Dazhui (GV 14) and Quchi (LI 11) eliminate heat and relieve exterior symptoms in obstruction syndrome with fever. Geshu (B 17) and Xuehai (Sp 10) promote circulation of blood in wandering syndrome, based on the principle that smooth blood circulation drives pathogenic wind away. The spleen controls the four limbs and its disturbance in transportation and transformation will cause retention of water, which is considered the cause of fixed pain syndrome. Therefore, Shangqiu (Sp 5) and Zusanli (S 36) are used to strengthen the function of the spleen and stomach for the purpose of eliminating pathogenic dampness—the root cause of the disorder.

B. Cutaneous Needling and Cupping

Both sides of the vertebra or the local involved joints are tapped heavily with a plum-blossom needle until bleeding a little, followed by cupping. This is often useful for rheumatoid arthritis.

C. Point Injection

Inject any solution of Chinese angelica, the root of Chinese clematis or *Radix*

Ledebouriellae into the points on the shoulder, elbow, hip and knee joints. Each point is administered with 0.5 to 1 ml. Never inject the drug into the articular cavity. Treatment is given once every one to three days. Ten treatments make a course. It is not advisable to use too many points in one treatment. For cases of multiple arthrosis, key points are taken first, then other points are used in turn.

Remarks

(1) Acupuncture treatment is especially good for obstruction syndromes, but it is impossible to get good results in a short time in the treatment of rheumatoid arthritis.

(2) Correct diagnosis must be made between bone tuberculosis and bone tumour in order to avoid delay in treatment.

33. Atrophic Syndromes and Sequelae of Poliomyelitis

Atrophic syndromes are characterized by limb flaccidity, motor impairment, or muscular atrophy of the lower limbs. Atrophic syndromes are often seen in multiple neuritis, sequelae of poliomyelitis, acute myelitis, myasthenia gravis, hysterical paralysis and periodic paralysis.

Etiology and Pathology

Atrophic syndromes are caused by malnourishment of tendons and consumption of the lung fluid due to invasion of the lung by exogenous pathogenic wind and heat or by attack of the dampness and heat, on the Yangming meridians, or by malnourishment of tendons and loss of essence and qi of the liver and kidney, due to a long duration of an illness or sexual indulgence.

Differentiation

Symptoms of the disorders are muscular flaccidity and muscular atrophy of limbs with motor impairment, which are different from those due to a heavy sensation and pain in obstruction. In the beginning there is usually fever, followed by muscular flaccidity of the limbs, upper or lower, left or right. In severe cases the lower limbs cannot move at all; muscles get thinner day by day, yet no pain is present.

(1) Atrophic syndromes due to heat in the lungs are marked by fever, cough, irritability, thirst, scant brownish urine, red tongue with yellow coating, and thin, rapid pulse besides the general symptoms.

(2) Atrophic syndromes due to dampness and heat: The accompanying symptoms are a general heavy sensation, cloudy, turbid urine, stuffiness in the chest, a hot sensation in the soles of the feet, alleviated by cold, sticky yellow tongue coating, lingering rapid pulse.

(3) Atrophic syndromes due to insufficiency of essence in the liver and kidney: The accompanying symptoms are weakness of the lumbar region, seminal emission, prospermia, dizziness, blurring of vision, red tongue, thin, rapid pulse.

Treatment

Method: Main points are in the Yangming meridians. Points in the Hand-Yangming Meridian are taken when the disorders are in the upper limbs, while points in the Foot-Yangming Meridian are taken when the disorders are in the lower limbs. For cases with excessive heat in the lungs or with dampness and heat, needling is given with the reducing method and moxibustion is not applicable. Sometimes plum-blossom needling is employed. For cases with insufficiency of essence of the liver and kidney, the reinforcing method is used.

Prescriptions:

Upper limb: Jianyu (LI 15), Quchi (LI 11), Hegu (LI 4), Yangxi (LI 5).

Lower limb: Biguan (S 31), Liangqiu (S 34), Zusanli (S 36), Jiexi (S 4).

Heat in the lungs: Chize (L 5), Feishu (B 13).

Dampness and heat: Yinlingquan (Sp 9), Pishu (B 20).

Insufficiency of essence of liver and kidney: Ganshu (B 18), Shenshu (B 23), Xuanzhong (G 39), Yanglingquan (G 34).

Explanation: These prescriptions are based on the principle of exclusive selection of points in the Yangming meridians in treatment of the atrophic syndromes, as stated in the *Inner Classic of the Yellow Sovereign*. Points in the Yangming meridians of Hand and Foot are taken alternately. Yangming meridians are full of qi and blood. They control tendons. The reducing method should be applied to eliminate excessive heat. Moxibustion alone or combined with acupuncture is given after heat subsides. Chize (L 5) and Feishu (B 13) are used to dissipate heat in the lungs. Yinlingquan (Sp 9) and Pishu (B 20) are taken to remove dampness and heat, because the lungs dominate qi, control respiration and regulate water passage; the spleen governs transportation and transformation. Ganshu (B 18) and Shenshu (B 23) are used to activate qi and tonify essence of the liver and kidney, since the liver controls the tendons and the kidney dominates the production of marrow. Yanglingquan (G 34), one of the eight influential points dominating tendons, and Xuanzhong (G 39), one of the eight influential points dominating marrow, are selected to invigorate the tendons and bones.

Modification: For cases with fever, Dazhui (GV 14) is added.

Remarks

(1) A long course of treatment is needed for atrophic syndromes. Acupuncture-moxibustion therapy is good to some extent for atrophic syndromes.

(2) In order to determine the affected parts and causative factors, consultations and examinations are necessary. Medication, massage and physiotherapy as part of the treatment should be taken into consideration for more effective results.

It is essential to do some functional exercises under the guidance of a doctor.

Sequelae of poliomyelitis

Sequelae of poliomyelitis is also known as sequelae of infantile paralysis. It is an acute infectious viral disease, often occurring in summer and autumn in children aged one to five. At the acute stage clinical manifestations are headache, fever, sore throat, nausea, vomiting, etc., as usually found in acute febrile diseases. Atrophic syndromes are present only when limb paralysis appears. Here only limb paralysis is dealt with.

Limb paralysis usually occurs after subsidence of the acute symptoms. It lasts for one to two weeks and then begins to recover. Marked improvement is seen in six months, after which less progress is seen. Some cases can gradually recover in one or two years, but some never recover completely. Muscular flaccidity, atrophy, deformity of joints, characterized by weakness, thinness, a cold sensation and deformity in the lower limbs, remain.

Treatment

A. Body Acupuncture

Method: Main points are in the Yangming meridians of Hand and Foot, in association with points in the affected areas. The reducing and reinforing methods are applied according to individual cases. Electroacupuncture can be used too.

Prescription:

Paralysis of the lower limbs: Shenji (Jiaji point, at the second lumbar vertebra), Huantiao (G 30), Yinmen (B 37), Futu (S 32), Zusanli (S 36), Yanglingquan (G 34).

Modifications:

Difficulty in lifting legs: Biguan (S 31) and Jianxi (three cun above the upper margin of the patella) are added.

Flexion of knee: Yinshi (S 33) and Jianqi (Extra) are added.

Back flexion of knee: Chengfu (B 36), Weizong (B 40), Chengshan (B 57) are added.

Foot ptosis: Jingxia (three cun above Jiexi, one cun lateral to the external border of tibia) and Jiexi (St 41) are added.

Inversion of foot: Fengshi (GB 31), Kunlun (UB 60), Qiuxu (GB 40), Xuanzhong (GB 39) and Jiuneifan (one cun lateral to Chengshan, UB 57) are added.

Eversion of foot: Jixia (two cun below Jimen), Yanglingquan (G 34), Sanyinjiao (Sp 6), Taixi (K 3) and Jiuwaifan (one cun medial to Chengshan, B 57) are added.

Heel walking: Chengshan (B 57), Kunlun (B 60) and Taixi (K 3) are added.

Paralysis of the upper limb: Jiaji points in the neck region (0.5 cun lateral to posterior midline), Naoshu (SI 10), Jianyu (LI 15), Jianliao (TE 14), Quchi (LI 11), Shousanli (LI 10) and Hegu (LI 4) are added.

Modifications:

Difficulty in lifting arm: Tianzong (SI 11), Jubi (three and a half cun inferior and anterior to the acromion), Binao (LI 14).

Failure in extension and flexion of elbow: Hongzhong (two and a half cun below Tianquan, S 25), Bizhong (Extra 32), Neiguan (P 6), Waiguan (TE 5).

Intorsion and extorsion of hand: Yangchi (TE 4), Yangxi (LI 5), Houxi (SI 3), Sidu (TE 9), Shaohai (H 3).

Wrist drop: Waiguan (TE 5), Sidu (TE 9).

Paralysis of abdominal muscles: Jiaji, Liangmen (S 21), Tianshu (S 25), Daimai (G 26).

Custaneous needling can be used in the local area in combination with the points.

B. Point Injection

Main and secondary points are taken as above.

Method: 10 percent glucose solution, vitamin B_1, fursultiamine hydrochloride, Chinese angelica compound solution, vitamin B_{12}, galanthaminum solution are administered. The 10 percent glucose solution must be injected into the spastic muscle group, such as points of Yinmen (B 37), Futu (S 32), Zusanli (S 36), etc.—10 ml solution for each point. Doses for other infections depend on the disease condition. For cases of mild paralysis one ampoule is enough, but for severe cases two ampoules are administered. Two to four points are taken for each treatment; 0.5 to 1 ml is injected into each point. Treatment is given once daily or every other day. Ten to twenty treatments make up a course.

C. Suture-embedding Therapy

See prescriptions for acupuncture mentioned above.

Remarks

In recent years oral live polio virus vaccine has been administered to prevent the occurrence of this disease. Sequelae of poliomyelitis should be treated promptly, combined with physical therapy. For severe joint deformity, orthopedic operation may be considered.

34. Polyneuritis

Polyneuritis is also known as terminal (peripheral) neuritis, characterized by symmetrization, sensory disturbance of the distal ends of the extremities and relaxant paralysis. It is usually caused by infection, poisoning, metabolic disturbance and genetic or allergic factors.

In early stages symptoms are pain in limbs, numbness from invasion of the tendons by pathogenic dampness and obstruction of meridians. In late stages consumption of essence and blood due to heat from accumulated dampness appears. When the tendons are unnourished, numbness and weakness of the limbs and muscular atrophy may occur. These belong to the atrophic syndromes.

Differentiation

Early-stage symptoms are numbness of fingers and toes, stabbing pain, paresthesia and allergy, followed by sensory disturbances. In a typical case manifestations are sensory trouble in the ends of the four limbs, as though they were wearing gloves and socks, attenuating or disappearing, relaxant paralysis in the distal ends of limbs, weakness in movement, muscular atrophy leading to ptosis of wrist or ptosis of foot, disappearance of tendon reflex, smooth, thin skin in the affected regions, cold sensation, hidrosis or lack of hidrosis.

Treatment

A. Body Acupuncture

Method: Main points are in the Yangming meridians of Hand and Foot and adjacent points. Needling is given with the reinforcing method.

Prescription: Jianyu (LI 15), Quchi (LI 11), Hegu (LI 4), Huantiao (G 30), Yanglingquan (G 34), Zusanli (S 36), Xuanzhong (G 39), Sanyinjiao (Sp 6).

Explanation: The prescription is still based on the principle of selecting points of the Yangming meridians to treat atrophic syndromes. Jianyu (LI 15), Quchi (LI 11), Shousanli (LI 10), Hegu (LI 4) and Zusanli (S 36) are prescribed to regulate qi and blood and nourish tendons. Waiguan (TE 5), Huantiao (G 30), Yanglingquan (G 34), Xuanzhong (G 39) and Sanyinjiao (Sp 6) are used in combination. Among them Huantiao (G 30) can regulate qi flow of the body and invigorate the qi and blood in the lower limbs. Yanglingquan (G 34), one of the eight influential points dominating tendons, is for readjusting the functions of tendons. Xuanzhong (G 39), one of the eight influential points dominating marrow, combined with Yanglingquan (G 34) is used with the reinforcing method for replenishing marrow and strengthening tendons and bones. Sanyinjiao (Sp 6) is used to strengthen the function of the spleen and eliminate dampness. In addition, according to the disease conditions, some other points can also be chosen, e.g. Yangchi (TE 4) and Shaohai (H 3) in the upper limbs and Fengshi (G 31), Qiuxu (G 40) and Bafeng (Extra 36), etc., in the lower limbs.

B. Point Injection

Method: Any solution of 0.5 ml of vitamin B_1, B_6, B_{12} is injected into each point. Two points are selected for each treatment once every other day. Ten treatments make up a course.

C. Cutaneous Needling

Method: Cutaneous needling is applied to the endings of fingers and toes or the affected areas. Scattered tapping is done from the proximal to distal along the running course of the channels around the affected areas. The therapy can also be applied to the back of the head. Treatment is given once a day or every other day. Thirty treatments constitute a course.

Remarks

Attention should be paid to the cause of the disease. A long period of treatment is advised because of slow recovery. For cases with motor impairment assign physiotherapy, physical exercise therapy and functional exercises.

35. Facial Paralysis

Facial paralysis is the weakening or paralysis of facial nerves, as in Bell's palsy. Peripheral facial paralysis is often seen in clinical practice. It occurs in people of any age, but most patients are between twenty and forty, male outnumbering female.

The causative factors are constant muscular relaxation resulting from invasion of the Yangming and Shaoyang meridians by pathogenic wind and cold, obstruction of meridians and failure of the tendons to be nourished.

Differentiation

Facial paralysis occurs suddenly. Upon waking, one finds regidity, numbness and paralysis of one side of the face, inability to frown, raise the eyebrows, open the mouth and blow out the cheek, deviation of the mouth towards the healthy side, incomplete closing of the eyes, lacrimation, disappearance of frontal striae, shallow nasolabial groove on the affected side. In some cases there may be pain in the back or the inferior region of the ear and face in the beginning. In severe cases two thirds of the tongue on the affected side may lose its sense of taste, and hyperacusia may occur also.

Treatment

A. Body Acupuncture

Method: Main points are in the Yangming meridians of Hand and Foot, supplemented by points in the Shaoyang and Taiyang meridians of Hand and Foot. Local and distal points along the meridians are usually needled, the former punctured superficially and horizontally towards another point or obliquely.

Prescription: Fengchi (G 20), Yangbai (G 14), Zanzhu (B 2), Sibai (S 2), Dicang (S 4), Hegu (LI 4), Taichong (Liv 3).

Modifications:

For cases with shallow nasolabial groove, Yingxiang (LI 20) is added.

For cases with deviation of the philtrum groove, Shuigou (GV 26) is added.

For cases with deviation of the mentolabial groove, Chengjiang (CV 24) is added.

For cases with pain in the mastoid region, Yifeng (TE 17) is added.

Explanation:

Fengchi (G 20) and Yifeng (TE 17), pertaining to the Shaoyang meridians, are taken to eliminate pathogenic wind; Yifeng (TE 17) can both eliminate wind and relieve pain. It is helpful in treatment of pain in the mastoid region. Yangbai (G 14), Zanzhu (B 2), Sibai (S 2) and Dicang (S 4) are used to regulate the meridian qi. These points are selected according to the paralytic location. The technique of horizontal penetration of two points may be used to enhance the effect of regulating the meridian qi; for example, you may needle Dicang (S 4) horizontally towards Jiache (S 6). Hegu (LI 4) and Taichong (Liv 3), the two distal points along the course of the meridian are used to relieve disorders in the head and face.

B. Point Injection

Method: Solution of vitamin B_1 or vitamin B_{12} is injected into Yifeng (TE 17) and Qianzheng (Extra), 0.5 to 1 ml for each point. Treatment is given daily or every other day. The above points can be used alternately.

C. Electroacupuncture

Method: Select points in the facial region; after needle insertion, the current is turned on for five to ten minutes until the paralytic muscles contract. Treatment is given daily or every other day.

D. Cutaneous Needling

Method: Cutaneous needling is used to prick Yangbai (G 14), Taiyang (Extra 2), Sibai (S 2) and Qianzheng until bleeding slightly, then cupping is applied for five to ten minutes. Treatment is given every other day.

It is helpful for an incipient condition or sensation of rigidity in the facial region or sequelae of facial paralysis.

E. Point Compress

Method: 10 to 20 g Strychnos Nux-Vomica powder is applied externally to Xiaguan (S 7), dressed with a piece of adhesive tape, for two to three days. Four or five applications make up a course.

Remarks

(1) It is essential to make a correct diagnosis for peripheral or central-nervous-

system facial paralysis.

(2) In the incipient stage do not use strong stimulation in acupuncture. Avoid wind and cold. During treatment, massage and hot compress to the facial region are helpful. Eye shades or eyedrops are used to keep away infection of the eyes.

36. Sciatica

Sciatica refers to pain anywhere along the course of the sciatic nerves, caused by various factors.

Etiology and Pathology

The condition includes primary sciatic neuralgia (sciatic neuritis), which is related to wind and dampness, infection, and affection of cold, and secondary sciatic neuralgia, which is caused by mechanical pressure or adhesion due to disorders of proximal tissues of the nerve course, such as prolapse of the intervertebral disc, tumour of the spine, TB or pathological changes at articulations intervertebrales, sacroiliac joints and pelvis, and injury to soft tissues in the lumbosacral region. Depending on the lesion, there is nerve-root sciatica or nerve-trunk sciatica. In "Treatise on Total Obstruction Syndromes, Miraculous Pivot" it says that pathogenic wind, cold and dampness lodge between the subcutaneous tissues and muscles, causing pain to run up and down the meridians and preventing the body from turning left and right. It is the earliest description of this condition in ancient medical classics.

Differentiation

Sciatica is manifested by paroxysmal or persistent burning or stabbing pain radiating from the back to the buttocks and lower limbs along their back and sides, aggravated when walking. Straight-leg lifting test is positive.

The onset of primary sciatica is an acute or subacute condition. Radiating pain and markedly tender spots appear along the courses of the sciatic nerves. There is sharp pain a few days after the onset, but the pain is gradually relieved in several weeks or months. Relapse is often induced by affection of cold-dampness.

Cases of secondary attack often have a history of primary sciatica. Pain is aggravated on coughing, sneezing or bowel movement. There are tenderness and pain on percussion in the side of the lumbar vertebra, motor impairment of the lumbar region and pain radiating to the lower limbs upon movement.

Treatment

A. Body Acupuncture

Method: Main points are in the Taiyang and Shaoyang meridians of Foot. Generally, needling is done with the reducing method, combined with moxibustion or cupping.

Prescription: Shenshu (B 23), Dachangshu (B 25), Jiaji points from the second to the fifth lumbar vertebra, Zhibian (B 54), Huantiao (G 30), Yinmen (B 37), Weizhong (B 40), Chengshan (B 57), Yanglingquan (B 34), Juegu (G 39).

Explanation: Shenshu (B 23), Dachangshu (B 25), Zhibian (B 54) and Huantiao (G 30) are taken since the lesions are located between the vertebral and gluteal regions. Deeper needling is applied to the Jiaji points to make the needle sensation go downwards, eliminating the pathogenic factors and obstruction of the meridians. Yinmen (B 37), Weizhong (B 40), Changshan (B 57), Yanglingquan (G 34) and Juegu (G 39) are located where the radiating pain occurs. The reducing method is applied to these points to alleviate pain. For incipient cases with sharp pain due to obstruction of the meridians, distal points can be also used. Sometimes piercing needling is given to Yemen (TE 2) horizontally towards Zhongzhu (TE 3) to remove disorders. If intolerance to cold and preference for warmth occur in the diseased part, moxibustion or cupping is advisable to Yanglingquan (G 34) and Zusanli (S 36), so pathogenic wind, cold and dampness can be driven away.

B. Point Injection

Method: Prepare a 10 percent glucose solution of 10 to 20 ml and add vitamin B_1 (100 mg) or vitamin B_{12} (100 mg). Inject 5 to 10 ml into each of the Jiaji points from the second to the fourth lumbar vertebra and Zhibian (B 54). Two or three points are used each time. When the strong needling sensation extends downward to the leg, raise the needle a bit and quickly inject the drug. Treatment is given once every other day. For cases with sharp pain 5 to 10 ml of 10 percent procaine solution is injected into Huantiao (G 30) or Ahshi points.

C. Electroacupuncture

Main points:

Nerve-root sciatica: Jiaji points from the fourth to fifth lumbar vertebra, Yanglingquan (G 34), Weizhong (B 54).

Nerve-trunk sciatica: Zhibian (B 54) or Huantiao (G 30), Yanglingquan (G 34) or Weizhong (B 54).

Method: Use relatively strong high-frequency stimulation for five to ten minutes.

D. Ear Acupuncture

Main points: Sciatic Nerve, Adrenal, Buttocks, Ear Shenmen, Lumbar Vertebrae, Sacrum.

Method: Moderate or strong stimulation is applied. The needles are retained for ten to thirty minutes with twirling every five minutes. Treatment is given once a day or every other day. Needle embedding for three to seven days is sometimes used.

Remarks

(1) If sciatica is caused by a tumour or tuberculosis, treat the primary disease. Manipulation and massage are applied with acupuncture for sciatica due to prolapse of the intervertebral disc.

(2) At the acute stage patients are advised to stay in bed. Patients with prolapse of the intervertebral disc must lie on a hard bed.

(3) Keep warm. Maintain good posture or fasten a wide belt around waist during manual labour.

37. Trigeminal Neuralgia

Trigeminal neuralgia refers to an excruciating episodic pain in the facial area around the trigeminal nerve. There are primary and secondary conditions. The problem usually occurs in middle-aged people, especially females.

Etiology and Pathology

Causative factors are not clear up to now. It is generally held that a primary case is related to affection of cold, viral infection and tooth disease, and a secondary case may be caused by the impact of tumour pressure, inflammation and deformity of blood vessels.

Differentiation

Pain suddenly attacks the area around the trigeminal nerve, often in the maxillary and mandibular region (the second and third branches) and seldom in the opthalmic region (the first branch). Rarely are three branches on one side or both sides involved simultaneously. The pain lasts a very short time, a few seconds or minutes. Relapse occurs in several hours or days when a certain point on the face is touched, so patients are afraid to wash their face, brush their teeth and eat food. The transient, paroxysmal, sharp pain is accompanied by muscle spasm, uncontrollable tears, runny nose and saliva on the affected side. Generally, primary trigeminal neuralgia has no marked positive phenomena of the nervous system. The attack is episodic. If there is other injury to the nerve system or aggravated persistent paroxysmal pain, secondary trigeminal neuralgia, caused by intracranial disorders, should be considered.

Treatment

A. Body Acupuncture

Method: Local and distal points along the course of the meridians are selected. The reducing method is used with continuous needle twirling.

Prescriptions:

Point location / Branch	Local points		Distal points
Pain along the first (ophthalmic) branch	Zanzhu (B 2), Yangbai (G 14), Yuyao (Extra 3)		
Pain along the second (maxillary) branch	Sibai (S 2), Nose Juliao (S 3) Quanliao (SI 18)	Xiaguan (S 7)	Hegu (LI 4) Sanjian (LI 3) Neiting (S 44)
Pain along the third (mandibular) branch	Jiachengjiang (Extra), Jiache (S 6)		

Explanation: Points are selected according to the affected area and branch, e.g. Zanzhu (B 2), Sibai (S 2) and Jiachengjiang (Extra), located in the region around the trigeminal nerve, are taken to regulate the meridian qi in the affected area. When the qi flows smoothly, the pain stops. Hegu (LI 4), Sanjian (LI 3) and Neiting (S 44), pertaining to the Yangming meridians of Hand and Foot, which pass through the cheeks, are used to regulate the qi of the individual channels. This is known as "selecting points of the lower part for disorders of the upper."

B. Ear Acupuncture

Method: Select two or three points for each treatment. Needles are retained for twenty to thirty minutes with needle twirling every five minutes or needles embedded in the points.

(3) Point Injection

Method: Inject vitamin B_{12}, vitamin B_1 or procaine solution into the tender spots injecting 0.5 to 1 ml into each point. Treatment is applied once every two or three days.

Remarks

Acupuncture treatment can alleviate trigeminal neuralgia. It is essential to determine the cause of the secondary trigeminal neuralgia or trigeminal nerve paralysis. Appropriate measures are taken accordingly.

38. Menstrual Irregularities

Irregularities include abnormalities in the cycle, amount and colour of menstrual flow and other symptoms. Clinically, early and late menstruations are common.

Etiology and Pathology

Early menstruation usually results from anxiety leading to stasis of qi. Long-standing qi may turn into fire in the uterus. Abundant heat disturbs the normal flow of blood and menstruation comes ahead of time. Late menstruation is usually caused by invasion of the uterus by pathogenic cold or by insufficient blood and yang deficiency, which impairs the function of the Chong and Conception Vessel meridians. Menoxenia usually results from excessive childbearing, sexual indulgence, long-standing hemorrhagic disorders and deficiency in the spleen and stomach or impairment of the liver and kidney.

Differentiation

(1) Early menstruation comes earlier than expected or even twice a month. Menstrual flow is bright red or purple, accompanied by a feverish sensation, thirst, preference for cold beverages, rapid pulse, red tongue with yellow coating.

(2) Late menstruation comes later than the due time or once every forty to fifty days. The menstrual flow is light red, accompanied by aversion to cold, slow pulse and pale tongue.

(3) Menoxenia is irregular menstruation with excessive or scant dark-red or light-red menstrual flow. Weak constitution, sallow complexion, thin, slow pulse, and pale tongue may also appear.

Treatment

A. Body Acupuncture

Method: Main points are in the Conception Vessel and Foot-Taiyin meridians. Early menstruation is treated only by acupuncture without moxibustion. Needling is given with the half reinforcing, half reducing method. Acupuncture and moxibustion are employed for late menstruation or menoxenia.

Prescription: Qihai (CV 6), Sanyinjiao (Sp 6).

Modifications:

Early menstruation: Taichong (Liv 3) and Taixi (K 3) are added. Late menstruation: Xuehai (Sp 10) and Guilai (S 29) are added.

Menoxenia: Shenshu (B 23), Jiaoxin (K 8), Pishu (B 20) and Zusanli (S 36) are added.

Explanation: The treatment aims at regulating the function of the Chong and Conception Vessel meridians and smoothing the flow of qi and blood. The Conception

Vessel Meridian controls the uterus. When its qi is sufficient, menstruation will be normal. Qihai (CV 6) is taken to reinforce the body's primary qi. Since the qi governs the blood, sufficient qi controls the normal flow of blood. The spleen and stomach are the source of blood formation. If there is plenty of qi in the spleen, blood will be well governed. Therefore Sanyinjiao (Sp 6) is used in combination. For cases of early menstruation due to heat in the blood, Taichong (Liv 3) is added to eliminate heat in the liver. Taixi (K 3) is added to replenish the kidney yin and regulate menstruation. Late menstruation due to stasis of blood should be treated by needling Xuehai (Sp 10), Guilai (S 29) and Qihai (CV 6) with the reducing method to promote circulation of qi and blood. If it is caused by insufficiency of blood, acupuncture and moxibustion may be used together to warm up the meridians and enrich blood. Menoxenia is due to deficiency of inborn kidney qi and of acquired qi and blood. That is why Shenshu (B 23) and Jiaoxin (K 8) are used to replenish the kidney qi. Pishu (B 20) and Zusanli (S 36) are selected to help the middle burner provide qi and blood.

B. Ear Acupuncture

Main points: Uterus, Endocrine, Ovary, Kidney, Liver.

Method: Two or three points are selected for each treatment. Needles are manipulated with moderate or strong stimulation and retained for fifteen to twenty minutes. Needle embedding may also be used.

C. Suture-embedding Therapy

Method: A piece of 1 cm sterilized catgut is embedded subcutaneously at Sanyinjiao (Sp 6) or Zhongji (CV 3) towards Guanyuan (CV 4) before or after the menstrual period, causing the therapeutic result to last longer.

Remarks

(1)Hygiene should be observed during the menstrual period; avoid cold, raw or pungent food, mental irritation and heavy physical labour.

(2) Acupuncture treatment is usually given three to five days before menstruation. Three to five treatments are administered in succession. Another course of treatment is not given until the next period.

39. Dysmenorrhea

Dysmenorrhea refers to severe pain in the lower abdomen prior to, during or after the menstruation period.

Etiology and Pathology

The condition may be a deficient or excessive type. Dysmenorrhea of the excessive type is usually caused by affection by cold during menstruation, leading to retardation of blood in the uterus. Failure of normal menstrual flow is the cause of dysmenorrhea. It may also be the result of emotional depression and stagnation of qi. Dysmenorrhea of the deficient type is usually caused by a weak constitution or insufficiency of blood after a serious illness or long-standing disease. Insufficient blood in the uterus and malnourishment of the vessels lead to dysmenorrhea.

Differentiation

Main complaint is lower abdominal pain during, before or after menstruation.

(1) Dysmenorrhea of the excessive type is manifested by abnormal menstrual flow, lower abdominal pain, aggravated by pressure, purple menstrual flow with clotting, pain relieved after the clots are removed, deep, retarded pulse. Sometimes a distending sensation radiates to the costal and hypochondriac region in addition to pain, fullness in the chest, nausea, and taut pulse.

(2) Dysmenorrhea of the deficient type is marked by insidious and persistent abdominal pain after menstruation, alleviated by pressure and warmth, scant menstruation, lassitude in the lower back and limbs, poor appetite, dizziness, palpitation, thin, weak pulse, and pale tongue.

Treatment

A. Body Acupuncture

a. Dysmenorrhea of the excessive type

Method: Main points are in the Conception Vessel and Foot-Taiyin meridians. Needling is done with the reducing method. Moxibustion may also be applied.

Prescription: Zhongji (CV 3), Ciliao (B 32), Diji (Sp 8).

Explanation: The main purpose of this prescription is to regulate the function of the Chong and Conception Vessel meridians and remove stagnated blood in order to stop pain. Zhongji (CV 3) is chosen to adjust the qi in the Chong and Conception Vessel meridians. Diji (Sp 8), the Xi (cleft) point of the Spleen Meridian, is used to regulate the qi in the Spleen Meridian and stop pain. Ciliao (B 32) is an empirical point for treating dysmenorrhea.

b. Dysmenorrhea of the deficient type

Method: Main points are in Conception Vessel, Governor Vessel Foot-Shaoyin and Yangming meridians. Needling is done with the reinforcing method. Moxibustion may also be applied.

Prescription: Mingmen (GV 34), Shenshu (B 23), Guanyuan (CV 4), Zusanli (S 36), Dahe (K 2).

Explanation: Points in this prescription are mainly used to regulate and invigorate qi and blood and warm up and nourish the Chong and Conception Vessel meridians. Mingmen (GV 34), dominating the yang meridians of the body, is chosen to refresh the kidney yang. Application of moxibustion to Shenshu (B 23), Back Shu points of the kidney and Dahe (K 12) can warm up and strengthen the kidney yang. Moxibustion applied to Guanyuan (CV 4) will warm up the lower burner and nourish the Governor Vessel and Conception Vessel meridians. Furthermore, Zusanli (S 36) will strengthen the function of the spleen and stomach and replenish qi and blood. If there is enough blood and qi to nourish the uterine vessels, the Chong and Conception Vessel meridians will work smoothly and harmoniously.

Modification: Guilai (S 29), Pishu (B 20), Sanyinjiao (Sp 6), and Taichong (Liv 3) may be added to this prescription.

B. Ear Acupuncture

Main points: Uterus, Endocrine, Sympathetic Nerve, Kidney.

Method: Two to four points are punctured with moderate or strong stimulations for each treatment. Needles are retained for fifteen to twenty minutes or embedded in the ear.

C. Point Injection

Method: one ml of 1 percent procaine is injected subcutaneously into Shangliao (B 31) and Ciliao (B 32). Treatment is given once a day.

D. Suture-embedding Therapy

Method: See "Menstrual Irregularities."

Remarks

a. Hygiene should be observed during menstruation. Avoid mental irritation, cold or overintake of raw and cold food.

b. Dysmenorrhea has various causes. Gynecologic examinations should be given to ensure correct diagnosis.

40. Amenorrhea

Amenorrhea occurs when menstruation has not begun by the age of eighteen or menstruation ceases for more than three months for causes other than pregnancy and breast feeding.

Etiology and Pathology

The condition includes deficient and excessive types. Causative factors are excessive childbearing, anxiety, weak constitution, or debility due to a long illness, resulting in functioned disturbance of the spleen and stomach in transportation and transformation and excessive consumption of blood. It is believed that a scanty blood source leads subsequently to amenorrhea. Sometimes it is caused by cold affection that lodges in the uterus or by mental depression, stagnation of qi and stasis of blood and obstruction of the channels.

Differentiation

Amenorrhea is due either to exhaustion of blood or blood stasis.

(1) Exhaustion of blood is manifested by menstrual flow decreasing in amount to menstrual stoppage, usually accompanied by poor appetite, loose stool, pallor, dizziness, palpitation, lassitude, thin retarded pulse, pale tongue.

(2) Blood stasis symptoms are the cessation of menstruation, pain in the lower abdomen, a feverish sensation in the palms and soles, and fullness in the chest. In severe cases there may be swelling in the abdomen, constipation, dryness of the skin and mouth, dark-red tongue (with purple spots), deep, taut and retarded pulse.

Treatment

A. Body Acupuncture

a. Exhaustion of blood

Method: Points in the Conception Vessel Meridian and Back-Shu points are mainly selected. Needling is done with the reinforcing method. Moxibustion may also be applied.

Prescription: Pishu (B 20), Shenshu (B 23), Qihai (CV 6), Zusanli (S 36).

Explanation: The treatment aims at regulating the function of the spleen and stomach to enrich the kidney qi. The spleen and stomach are known as the material basis of the acquired constitution, dominating digestion, transforming the essences of food into qi and blood. Sufficient blood brings about normal menstruation, therefore Pishu (B 20) and Zusanli (S 36) are used to strengthen the function of the spleen and stomach. The kidney is thought to be the source of the inborn constitution. If its qi is sufficient, the essence of the kidney and blood will be ample, so Shenshu (B 23) and Qihai (CV 6) are chosen to enrich the qi of the kidney.

b. Stasis of blood

Method: Points are chiefly selected from the Conception Vessel, Foot-Taiyin and Jueyin meridians. Needling is given with the reducing method. Usually, moxibustion is not applied.

Prescription: Zhongji (CV 3), Hegu (LI 4), Xuehai (Sp 10), Sanyinjiao (Sp 6) and Xingjian (Liv 2).

Explanation: Points in this prescription can eliminate heat and promote production of fresh blood. Zhongji (CV 3) regulates the function of the Chong and Ren channels and the lower burner. Xuehai (Sp 10) and Xingjian (Liv 2) used in combination, regulate the qi in the liver and spleen and remove stagnation of qi and blood. Hegu (LI 4) and Sanyinjiao (Sp 6) make the qi and blood descend and produce normal menstruation.

B. Ear Acupuncture

Main points: Endocrine, Liver, Kidney, Spleen, Ear Shenmen, Subcortex.

Method: Treatment is given every other day with moderate stimulation. Ten treatments make up a course.

Remarks

Amenorrhea should be differentiated from early pregnancy. It is necessary to have an appropriate examination before acupuncture treatment in order to determine the causative factors and take timely corresponding medical measures.

41. Uterine Bleeding

Excessive uterine bleeding outside the regular menstruation period or incessant dripping of blood, sudden profuse uterine bleeding or mild, persistent vaginal bloody discharge, may lead into one another. In some cases the former syndrome, if not treated by emergency measures, may transform into the latter syndrome, while the latter may transform into the former if it is prolonged.

Etiology and Pathology

Causative factors are impairment of the Chong and Conception Vessel meridians and dysfunction of the liver and spleen. The kidney controls storage of essence, and sexual indulgence injures the kidney and Chong and Conception Vessel meridians. Eventually they fail to control the blood vessels. Other causes are mental depression resulting in dysfunction of the liver, retardation of qi and blood and production of heat, leading to uterine bleeding. Sometimes it is caused by irregular food intake or long-standing anxiety, which weakens the spleen in control of blood.

Differentiation

The nature of the disease—cold, heat, deficiency and excess—is differentiated on the basis of menstrual quantity, consistency, colour, and smell, pulse and tongue condition, general symptoms and signs.

(1) Heat syndromes due to excessive pathogenic factors: Manifested by discharge of profuse thick, offensive, purple blood with abdominal pain intensified by pressure, constipation, thirst, taut, rapid and strong pulse, red tongue with yellow coating.

(2) Yin deficiency syndromes: Marked by discharge of bright-red blood, dizziness, tinnitus, palpitation, insomnia, afternoon fever, thin, rapid and weak pulse.

(3) Qi deficiency syndromes: Characterized by continual uterine bleeding, discharge of red blood, cold sensation and pain in the lower abdomen, pallor, lassitude, listlessness, somnolence, poor appetite slow, thin pulse.

(4) Collapse syndrome: Continual scanty or sudden profuse uterine bleeding, syncope, pallor, cold sweating, shortness of breath, cold limbs, thin, fading pulse.

Treatment

A. Body Acupuncture

Method: Main points are in the Conception Vessel and Foot-Taiyin meridians. Needling is done with the reducing method for heat syndromes. Moxibustion is not advisable. The reinforcing method is used for deficiency and cold syndromes. Moxibustion should be applied often.

Prescription: Guanyuan (CV 4), Sanyinjiao (Sp 6), Yinbai (Sp 1).

Heat syndromes: Xuehai (Sp 10) and Shuiquan (K 5).

Yin deficiency syndromes: Neiguan (P 6) and Taixi (K 3).

Qi deficiency syndromes: Pishu (B 20) and Zusanli (S 36).

Collapse syndromes: Baihui (GV 20) and Qihai (CV 6).

Explanation: This prescription regulates and reinforces the qi in the Chong and Conception Vessel meridians and eliminates heat and stagnation of blood. Guanyuan (CV 4), as a point where the three foot yin meridians and Chong and Conception Vessel meridians meet, invigorates their qi and controls blood flow. Sanyinjiao (Sp 6), the crossing point of the three foot yin meridians strengthens the function of the spleen and controls blood. This is considered a key point in treating gynecological illnesses. Yinbai (Sp 1), the Jing (Well) point of the Spleen Meridian, is commonly used in treating uterine bleeding.

Modification: For cases with abundant heat, Xuehai (Sp 10) and Shuiquan (K 5) are used to eliminate heat in the blood and check bleeding. For cases with qi deficiency, Zusanli (S 36) and Pishu (B 20) are added to replenish the qi of the middle burner and control blood. For cases with yin deficiency, Neiguan (P 6) and Taixi (K 3) are added to adjust the function of the heart and kidney and clear off heat due to deficiency. Moxibustion applied to Baihui (GV 20) and Qihai (CV 6) refreshes the primary qi, rescues collapsing yang and revives the patient.

B. Scalp Acupuncture

Bilateral reproductive regions are selected. Twirl the needles for three to five minutes. A second twirling of the needles is given after an interval of five minutes, then a third.

C. Ear Acupuncture

Main points: Uterus, Subcortex, Endocrine, Ovary, Adrenal.

Method: Sensitive spots on the ear are taken first. Needles are retained for one to two hours with intermittent manipulation.

Remarks

(1) A menopausal woman suffering from repeated uterine bleeding should have a gynecological examination for possibility of tumour.

(2) Emergency measures should be adopted promptly in case of collapse due to massive bleeding.

42. Morbid Leukorrhea

Whitish viscid discharge from the vagina and uterine cavity is often seen in vaginitis, cervicitis, pelivoperitonitis, cervical cancer, etc.

Etiology and Pathology

Causative factors are mostly dysfunction of the Conception Vessel Meridian and failure of the Dai Meridian to exert its controlling function, causing downward infusion of turbid dampness. Leukorrhea is also caused by dysfunction of the spleen and stomach in transportation and transformation due to irregular food intake and overstrain, leading to accumulated dampness moving downward. Sometimes mental depression and long stagnated qi of the liver will give rise to fire. Confrontation between blood and heat, then downward infusion of damp heat results in pinkish leukorrhea and pinkish leukorrhea mixed with white matter.

Differentiation

Generally speaking, whitish leukorrhea is the most common, followed by whitish-yellowish leukorrhea and pinkish leukorrhea. Morbid leukorrhea can be divided into damp-heat and damp-cold types.

(1) Damp-heat type is marked by foul smell, yellowish leukorrhea, constipation, scant yellow urine, weak, rapid pulse, sticky yellow tongue coating, or by pinkish leukorrhea, bitter taste in the mouth, dryness of throat, restlessness, feverish sensation in the palms and soles, palpitation, insomnia, irritability, taut, rapid pulse, yellow coated tongue.

(2) Damp-cold type is manifested by long-term dilute leukorrhea with the smell of raw meat, heaviness and pain in the lumbar region, dizziness, lassitude, poor appetite, loose stool, coldness in the abdomen, slow, weak or deep, slow pulse, smooth white tongue coating.

Treatment

A. Body Acupuncture

Method: Main points are in the Conception Vessel, Dai and Foot-Taiyin meridians. Damp-heat type should be treated with the reducing method without moxibustion, while damp-cold type should be treated with the half reinforcing, half reducing method, supplemented by moxibustion.

Prescription: Daimai (G 26), Baihuanshu (B 30), Qihai (CV 6), Sanyinjiao (Sp 6).

Modifications:

Prominent damp heat: Xingjian (Liv 2) and Yinlingquan (Sp 9) are added.

Prominent damp cold: Guanyuan (CV 4) and Zusanli (S 36) are added.

Explanation: This prescription is used to strengthen the function of the spleen and remove dampness and regulate and reinforce the qi in the Conception Vessel and Dai meridians. Daimai (G 26) is used to refresh its meridian qi. Baihuanshu (B 30) and Qihai (CV 6) are chosen to adjust the qi in the Conception Vessel and urinary-bladder meridians and remove the pathogenic dampness. Sanyinjiao (Sp 6), as a point where the three Foot Yin meridians meet, is taken to strengthen the function of the spleen, eliminate dampness and harmonize the liver and kidney. In treatment of cases with prominent dampness and heat, Xingjian (Liv 2) is added to dispel accumulated heat in the Liver Meridian, while Yinlingquan (Sp 9) is added to clear off damp heat in the Spleen Meridian. For cases with abundant dampness and cold moxibustion applied to Guanyuan (CV 4) and Zusanli (S 36) is not only to warm up the lower burner but to strengthen the function of the spleen and remove dampness. Prolonged moxibustion of the two points can strengthen the body constitution and invigorate body resistance against pathogenic factors.

B. Ear Acupuncture

Main points: Uterus, Ovary, Endocrine, Urinary Bladder, Kidney.

Method: Three to five points are chosen for each treatment. Needles are retained for fifteen to twenty minutes.

Remarks

(1) Acupuncture treatment is effective to some extent for morbid leukorrhea. Women who have yellowish or pinkish leukorrhea must have gynecological examinations.

(2) Observe hygiene of the external genitalia.

43. Prolonged Labour

Prolonged labour refers to labour prolonged beyond the ordinary eighteen-hour limit.

Etiology and Pathology

Prolonged labour is usually due to the primipara's mental stress or an early birth, causing an early flow of amniotic fluid and massive loss of blood. It may also be caused by a weak constitution and deficiency of qi and blood.

Differentiation

Prolonged labour is manifested by early flow of amniotic fluid, labour pains abating, inability of the baby to be delivered, general lassitude, deep, thin or irregular pulse.

Treatment

Method: Points are mainly selected from the Hand-Yangming and Foot-Taiyin meridians.

Prescription: Hegu (LI 4), Sanyinjiao (Sp 6), Zhiyin (B 67), Duyin (Extra).

Explanation: Hegu (LI 4), the source point of the Hand-Yangming Meridian, and Sanyinjiao (Sp 6), the point where the three Foot Yin meridians meet, are used to invigorate qi and regulate blood, thus promoting delivery. Zhiyin (B 67), the Jing (Well) point of the Foot-Taiyang Meridian, and Duyin (Extra) are both empirical points in promoting delivery. Applying moxibustion to them can induce childbirth.

Remarks

Acupuncture treatment is effective to induce labour. If prolonged labour is caused by deformity of the uterus or a narrow pelvis, other appropriate measures must be taken.

44. Lactation Insufficiency and Lactifuge Method

Lactation insufficiency means the secretion of milk after childbirth cannot meet an infant's needs.

Etiology and Pathology

There are two conditions, deficiency and excess. The deficiency type is manifested by insufficiency of milk secretion or no milk at all, no distending sensation in the breast, pallor, poor appetite, shortness of breath, loose stool, lustreless lips and nails, thin pulse, pale tongue. Symptoms of the excess type are nonsecretion of milk, distending sensation in the breast, mental depression, stiffness in the chest, constipation, scant deep-yellow urine.

Treatment

A. Body Acupuncture

Method: Main points are in the Foot-Yangming Meridian. The reinforcing method with moxibustion is given to cases of deficiency and the half reinforcing, half reducing method is applied to cases of excess.

Prescription: Rugen (S 18), Shanzhong (CV 17), Shaoze (SI 1).

Modifications:

a. Excess type: Qimen (Liv 14) is added.

b. Deficiency type: Pishu (B 20) and Zusanli (S 36) are added.

Explanation: The Foot-Yangming Meridian passes through the breasts, and Rugen (S 18) in this meridian is located in the breast region. Selection of this point can regulate the qi of Foot-Yangming Meridian and promote secretion of milk. Shanzhong (CV 17) is used to regulate qi and strengthen the function of Rugen (S 18) in promoting secretion of milk. Shaoze (SI 1) is an empirical point used to promote lactation.

B. Ear Acupuncture

Main points: Mammary Gland, Endocrine, Chest Adrenal.

Method: Locate the sensitive spots on the ear first, then puncture the selected points. Needles are twirled for minutes, or embed the needles for one to seven days.

Remarks

Patients are advised to take nourishing food and soup. Breast-feed properly.

Lactifuge method

Foot Linqi (B 41) and Guangming (G 37) are punctured first, followed by moxibustion for ten minutes. Treatment is given once a day. Three to five treatments make up a course.

45. Prolapse of Uterus

The falling of the uterus to a position lower than the level of the spina ischiadica or the protrusion of the uterus through the vaginal orifice is termed prolapse of uterus. This disorder often occurs among labouring women in the countryside and women of excessive childbearing.

Etiology and Pathology

Prolapse of uterus is caused by weak constitution, qi and blood deficiency and early physical labour after giving birth, or by impairment of qi through excessive childbearing, leading to failure to raise the uterus.

Differentiation

The patient feels an object falling to the vagina through the vaginal orifice. It is as large as a goose egg and reddish. Subjective symptoms are a bearing-down sensation, pain in the lower back, lassitude, weak pulse and pale tongue. Recurrent attacks are usually induced by overstrain, severe coughing, difficult defecation. If the condition is not treated promptly, it will not be cured.

Treatment

A. Body Acupuncture

Method: Main points are in the Conception Vessel and Governor Vessel meridians. Needling is done mostly with the reinforcing method. Needles are retained, often with moxibustion.

Prescription: Baihui (GV 20), Qihai (CV 6), Dahe (K 12), Weidao (G 28), Taichong (Liv 3), Zhaohai (K 6).

Explanation: The treatment aims at invigorating vital energy to hold the uterus in position. Baihui (GV 20) is located at the vertex It is selected according to the principle of treating the upper part for diseases of the lower and using raising methods to treat sinking disorders. Qihai (CV 6) is taken to enrich qi, strengthen the function of lifting and keeping internal organs in their normal positions. Weidao (G 28), pertaining to the Foot-Shaoyang Meridian, a crossing point of the Dai Meridian, is used to hold and keep the uterus in its normal position. Both the liver and kidney channels pass through the lateral lower abdomen and connect with the uterus. So Taichong (Liv 3), Zhaohai (K 6) and Dahe (K 12) are chosen to promote the function of liver and kidney.

B. Electroacupuncture

The main point chosen is the middle one in the line connecting the anterior and superior iliac spine and ischial tuberosity. Needles are inserted obliquely to form an angle of 45 degrees to the inguinal groove and directly to the uterus. The depth of needling is decided by the sensation of a back contracture of the uterus and a distending feeling in the lumbar region and vagina. The current is turned on for fifteen to twenty minutes. In cases of prolapse of the urinary bladder Qugu (CV 2) and Henggu (K 11) are added and needled perpendicularly 2.5 to 3 cun in depth. In cases of prolapse of the rectum the levator of the anus, 0.5 cun lateral to it, is punctured bilaterally 2 to 2.5 cun in depth until it produces a hot feeling and upward contracture of the anus. After each treatment patients are advised to do an exercise of sitting down and standing up with the feet crossed and to contract the anus.

C. Scalp Acupuncture

The foot motional region and the reproductive region are punctured bilaterally. Ten treatments make up a course. A second course follows after an interval of three to five days.

Remarks

The patient should avoid heavy physical labour and sexual activity during treatment and pay attention to hygiene to prevent secondary infections. The patient should contract and relax the anus alternately for ten to fifteen minutes twice a day.

46. Malposition of the Fetus

The fetus in an abnormal position in the uterus after a thirty-week pregnancy occurs frequently among multiparae or pregnant women with lax abdominal walls. Usually there are no subjective symptoms. Only obstetrical examinations show a breech or transverse position.

Treatment

Main point: Zhiyin (B 67).

Method: The patient is asked to loosen her belt and sit on a chair or lie on a bed. Moxibustion is applied to Zhiyin (B 67) bilaterally for fifteen to twenty minutes. The treatment is given once or twice a day until the fetus is in normal position.

An 80 percent success rate has been reported. The treatment is more helpful to multiparae than to primiparae. The most successful results were obtained in seven-month pregnancy: the treatment was less effective for eight-month or more pregnancy. Moxibustion is widely used, yet acupuncture may be applied to some cases.

Remarks

There are various causes of malposition of the fetus. It is necessary to make detailed examinations. If caused by narrowness of the pelvis and deformity of the uterus, other measures have to be taken.

47. Acute Infantile Convulsions

Spasm of the limbs, clenched jaws, and opisthotonos often occur in children below the age of three.

They are usually seen in infections of the central nervous system, such as epidemic cerebrospinal meningitis, Japanese encephalitis B and toxic desentery.

Etiology and Pathology

Acute infantile convulsions are due to a poor, weak constitution affected by exogenous pathogenic factors that intrude into the interior of the body along channels, causing inability of the body's yang to disperse and accumulation of excessive heat, finally leading to stirring of the wind of the liver. Sometimes they are due to irregular food intake, impairing the spleen and stomach in the function of distribution of the body fluid, leading to formation of phlegm that turns into heat and wind. They may also be caused by sudden fright.

Differentiation

Symptoms are manifested by high fever, flushed face, head shaking, gritting and grinding of the teeth, disturbed sleep, uncontrolled movements of the limbs, mental restlessness followed by coma, staring upward of the eyes, clenched jaws, opisthotonos, paroxysmal spasms and tremors of the four limbs, shortness of breath, constipation, deep-yellow urine, superficial, rapid, tense and taut pulse, dark-green and purple finger veins.

Treatment

A. Body Acupuncture

Method: Main points are in the Governor Vessel and Hand-Yangming meridians, secondary points in the Foot-Jueyin channel. Needling is done superficially without retention. The reducing method is used or points are pricked until bleeding. Moxibustion is not advisable.

Prescription: Shuigou (GV 26), Dazhui (GV 14), Hegu (LI 4), Shixuan (Extra 30), Yanglingquan (G 34), Taichong (Liv 3).

Explanation: Puncturing Shuigou (GV 26) regulates the Governor Vessel Meridian and helps the patient resuscitate. Dazhui (GV 14), a meeting point of the yang meridians, is used to disperse yang and eliminate pathogenic factors in the exterior of the body. Hegu (LI 4), the Yuan (Source) point of the large intestine, united with the lung in their functional yoke, disperses the qi in the lung and causes fever to subside. Pricking Shixuan (Extra 30) until bleeding is to drive pathogenic heat out of the channels and bring back consciousness. Convulsions are a violent involuntary contraction of tendons and muscles. Yanglingquan (G 34), the influential point of the tendons, is chosen to relax tendons. The liver dominates interior wind, therefore Taichong (Liv 3) is prescribed to reduce the wind in the liver, checking wind, eliminating heat, restoring consciousness and tranquilizing the mind.

Modification: In individual cases Quchi (LI 11) is added to reduce heat, while Yongquan (K 1) is added to reduce fire. Yintang (Extra 1) is added to eliminate heat and check fright. Fenglong (S 40) is added to resolve phlegm.

B. Ear Acupuncture

Main points: Sympathetic Nerve, Ear Shenmen, Subcortex, Brain Point, Heart.

Method: Strong stimulation is given in severe cases. Needles are retained for one hour.

Remarks

Acupuncture treatment is quite effective in relief of convulsions, but it is necessary to determine the cause and give appropriate treatment.

48. Chronic Infantile Convulsions and Sequelae of Encephalitis

Also known as chronic spleen convulsions in traditional Chinese medicine, chronic infantile convulsions are marked by spasm, emaciation, and diarrhoea. They are often seen in children below three years old, aggravated after a long or severe illness.

Etiology and Pathology

There are many causative factors for infantile convulsions such as typhoid fever, malaria, prolonged desentery or vomiting and diarrhoea, or the taking of too many cool or cold medicines, which impair the spleen and stomach, leading to invasion of the spleen by liver fire and interior stirring up of wind and contraction of tendons and muscles. Chronic convulsions may also be caused by prolonged acute infantile convulsions.

Differentiation

Symptoms are sallow complexion, emaciation, lassitude, weakness of the limbs, slack breathing, cold gas exhaled from the nose, poor appetite, metopism, lethargy with half-closed eyes, cold limbs, occasional vomiting, clear urine, loose stool or diarrhoea mixed with undigested food, intermittent neck rigidity and spasmodic limbs, deep, slow, weak pulse, pale tongue, pale finger veins.

Treatment

A. Body Acupuncture

Method: Points are mainly selected from the Conception Vessel and Foot-Yangming meridians. Needling is done with the reinforcing method, combined with moxibustion.

Prescription: Zhongwan (CV 12), Zhangmen (Liv 13), Qihai (CV 6), Tianshu (S 25), Zusanli (S 36), Xingjian (Liv 2).

Explanation: Selection of Zhongwan (CV 12), the influential point of the fu organs, and Zusanli (S 36), the He (Sea) point of the Foot-Yangming Meridian, is to tonify the spleen and stomach and benefit the acquired constitution. Zhangmen (Liv 13), the Front-Mu point of the spleen, is used to warm up and invigorate the spleen yang. Qihai (CV 6) is used to enrich the primary qi and promote the function of the spleen in transportation and transformation. Moxibustion applied to Tianshu (S 25), the Front-Mu point of the Large-Intestine Meridian, is to warm up the spleen and stomach, promote their functions in transportation and transformation and stop loose stools. Xingjian (Liv 2), the Xing (Spring) point of the liver channel, is taken to pacify the liver and check wind. In a word, this prescription warms and invigorates the spleen and stomach, enriching the primary qi and checking wind.

B. Cutaneous Needling

Main points: Dazhui (GV 12), Qihai (CV 6), Pishu (B 20), Huatuo Jiaji points from the T5 to L2.

Secondary points: Guanyuan (CV 4), Baihui (GV 20), Zhangmen (Liv 13), Tianshu (S 25).

Remarks

The symptoms of chronic infantile convulsions are similar to those of chronic meningitis. Acupuncture is used only to relieve symptoms and signs. The condition should be treated with medicinal herbs and Western drugs.

Sequelae of Encephalitis

Symptoms occurring in the restoration stage of Japanese encephalitis B, generally six months after the onset of encephalitis, are called the sequelae of encephalitis. Clinical manifestations are mental excitation and restlessness, dementia, aphasia, difficulty in swallowing, paralysis, contraction and tremor of the limbs.

Treatment

A. Body Acupuncture

Method: Treatment aims at tranquilizing the mind, promoting qi and blood circulation and removing obstruction of meridians. Local and distal points may be used in combination. Needling is done with the reducing method.

Prescriptions:

Mental excitation: Neiguan (P 6), Shenmen (H 7), Sanyinjiao (Sp 6), Anmian (Extra 8).

Dementia: Dazhui (GV 14), Yamen (GV 15), Fengchi (G 20), Baihui (GV 20).

Aphasia: Yamen (GV 15), Liangquan (CV 23), Guanchong (TE 1), Hegu (LI 4).

Difficulty in swallowing: Tiantu (CV 22), Liangquan (CV 23), Hegu (LI 4), Jiache (S 6).

Tremor: Shousanli (LI 10), Jianshi (P 5), Hegu (LI 4), Yanglingquan (G 34), Dazhui (GV 14), Anmian (Extra 8).

Paralysis of the limbs: See "Facial Paralysis" and "Apoplexy."

B. Scalp Acupuncture

Hemiplegia: Motional region of the healthy side. Tremor of the extremities: Chorea and Parkinsonism control region.

Aphasia: Speech Region.

Mental excitation and dementia: Mental and emotional region (2 cm, above the anterior hairline and 2 cm lateral to the midsagittal line of the head; should be punctured 2 cm deep, parallel to the midsagittal line).

Remarks

During acupuncture treatment functional exercises, such as intelligence training, speech training and other exercises for paralysed limbs, should be stressed. Massage may be applied in combination.

49. Infantile Malnutrition

Infantile malnutrition is a disorder usually found in children below the age of ten, characterized by pot belly, sparse hair, sallow, lustreless complexion, emaciation, etc. The causes may be malnutrition, irregular food intake, chronic diarrhoea, intestinal parasites and tuberculosis.

Etiology and Pathology

Infantile malnutrition is usually due to irregular food intake, early delactation, improper feeding, malnutrition after illness, overdose of cathartics and drastic purgatives or parasitic diseases, all of which may lead to impairment of the function of the spleen and stomach, exhaustion of body fluids, and retention of food. The retained food may turn to fire, and a prolonged case may develop into infantile malnutrition syndromes.

Differentiation

The condition develops gradually. In the beginning mild or afternoon fever, preference for savoury, salty and sour food, dryness in the mouth, pot belly, diarrhoea with foul smell, rice-water urine, restlessness, crying, loss of appetite, followed by retention of food, sallow complexion, scalely, dry skin, and sparse may appear. In prolonged cases there may be lassitude, weakness of the limbs, pallor, deep-red tongue, sticky yellow tongue coating or peeled tongue, taut and rapid or weak and soft pulse.

Treatment

A. Body Acupuncture

Method: Points are mainly selected from the Foot-Taiyin and Yangming Meridians. Superficial needling is given without retention of the needle and moxibustion. Prescription: Xiawan (CV 10), Zusanli (S 36), Shifeng (Extra 29), Shangqiu (Sp 5).

Explanation: The pathology of infantile malnutrition is nothing more than dysfunction of the spleen and stomach, which are believed the key part of the acquired constitution. Normal functioning of the spleen and stomach can transform air, food and water into qi, blood and other substances. That is why Xiawan (CV 10) is taken to harmonize the stomach and intestines and clear off fire. Zusanli (S 36), the He (Sea) point of the Foot-Yangming Meridian, is used to invigorate the function of the spleen and stomach. Shangqiu (Sp 5), the Jing (River) point of the Spleen Meridian, is selected to strengthen the spleen's function and remove retention of food and stagnation of qi. Shifeng (Extra 29) is pricked until a yellowish fluid flows. It is very effective in infantile malnutrition.

Modifications:

Parasitic disorder: Baichongwo (Extra) is added.

Afternoon fever: Dazhui (GV 14) is added.

The disease may also be treated by pricking Pishu (B 20), Weishu (B 21) and Ganshu (B 18).

B. Cutting Therapy

Method: Cut the skin vertically 0.4 cm where Yuji (L 10) is located and remove about 0.3 g fat, then dress the wound.

C. Cutaneous Needling

The back and sacral regions are tapped with a plum-blossom needle. Points on the limb may also be selected. Each treatment lasts ten to twenty minutes.

Remarks

(1) Regular meals should be given. Avoid overeating, hunger and greasy food.

(2) Appropriate nutrition should be given to babies after delactation.

(3) In case of infantile malnutrition due to intestinal parasites or tuberculosis, the primary affection must be treated first.

(4) Massage and chiropractic along the spine may also be applied.

50. Nocturnal Enuresis

Nocturnal enuresis means involuntary discharge of urine during sleep. It is usually seen in children. Any child over three unable to control urine discharge during sleep is considered to have a morbid state.

Etiology and Pathology

Normal urination depends upon smooth water metabolism of the kidney and the controlling function of the urinary bladder. If the qi in the kidney is insufficient and the urinary bladder fails to control urine, nocturnal enuresis occurs.

Differentiation

Manifestation is nocturnal enuresis during sleep. In mild cases enuresis occurs once in several nights, but in severe cases it occurs several times in one night. Lassitude, anorexia, emaciation and sallow complexion may appear in prolonged cases.

Treatment

A. Body Acupuncture

Method: Points from the Conception Vessel Meridian and Back-Shu points in the Urinary Bladder Meridian are mainly selected. Needling is done with the reinforcing method. Moxibustion may be applied.

Prescription: Guanyuan (CV 4), Zhongji (CV 3), Sanyinjiao (Sp 6), Shenshu (B 23), Pangguangshu (B 28).

Explanation: Main causes of this disease are qi deficiency and impairment of the water metabolism of the kidney. Therefore Guanyuan (CV 4) and Shenshu (B 23) are used to refresh the kidney qi and strengthen the lower burner. Sanyinjiao (Sp 6) is used to adjust the qi of the three yin meridians. As the lesion is in the urinary bladder, Pangguangshu (B 28) and Zhongji (CV 3) are used in combination to activate the vital function of the urinary bladder. This is called combining use of the Back-Shu and Front-Mu points.

B. Ear Acupuncture

Main points: Kidney, Urinary Bladder, Brain Point, Subcortex.

Method: Two or three points are punctured with moderate or strong stimulation. Needles are retained for ten to twenty minutes. Treatment is given every other day.

C. Point Injection

Method: One ml of 1 percent procaine is injected into Ciliao (UB 32) or Sanyinjiao (Sp 6). The two points are used alternately. Treatment is given every other day.

D. Scalp Acupuncture

Method: The foot mobility region is selected bilaterally. Needling is done by hand manipulation or current stimulation.

Remarks

(1) Acupuncture treatment is effective for nocturnal enuresis, but in cases of enuresis due to organic diseases, the primary affection should be treated first.

(2) During treatment the family should help the doctor by offering fewer drinks to the diseased child in the evening and waking him up in time to discharge urine. Encourage the diseased child to cultivate the habit of discharging urine actively and

dispel the sense of inferiority. Tell the child he should have full confidence to overcome the disease.

51. Erysipelas

Erysipelas is an acute contagious skin disease. The onset is followed by a sudden appearance of deep-red patches on the skin. In view of the affected areas there are different names for erysipelas in traditional Chinese medicine, i.e. head erysipelas, body erysipelas, or leg erysipelas.

Etiology and Pathology

This disease is caused by accumulated pathogenic damp heat in the spleen and stomach, which spreads to the legs and feet, or collection of heat poison in the blood or in the skin due to invasion by pathogenic wind and heat. Sometimes it is caused by a wound on the skin. Head erysipelas indicates affection by pathogenic wind-heat, while leg erysipelas suggests affection by damp heat.

Differentiation

Onset is abrupt; redness and swelling of the affected areas and burning pain, aggravated by pressure, spread quickly. Bright redness turns to a deep colour in the centre of the affected area. The condition disappears after desquamation several days later, or there are blisters, oozing ulcers, itching and pain, accompanied by irritability, thirst, fever, constipation, brownish urine. If there is high fever, vomiting, delirium and coma or occasional convulsions, it indicates invasion of the interior by the pathogenic heat poison.

Treatment

A. Body Acupuncture

Method: Main points are in the Foot-Yangming and Taiyin meridians. Puncture with the reducing method or prick until there is local bleeding.

Prescription: Hegu (LI 4), Quchi (LI 11), Zusanli (S 36), Jiexi (S 41), Yinlingquan (Sp 9), Xuehai (Sp 10), Weizhong (B 40), Ahshi points.

Explanation: The prescription is good for removing toxic wind heat and damp heat. Hegu (LI 4) and Quchi (LI 11) eliminate heat in the Yangming Meridian. Zusanli (S 36) and Jiexi (S 41), pertaining to the Stomach Meridian of Yangming, combined with Yinlingquan (Sp 9) of the Spleen Meridian of Foot-Taiyin, strengthen the function of the spleen and stomach so as to remove dampness and heat. Accumulated heat in the blood is removed by needling Xuehai (Sp 10) and Weizhong (B 40) and by pricking Ahshi points until bleeding. In traditional Chinese medicine "obstruction and stagnation of blood must removed."

B. Cupping and Bloodletting Therapy

Method: Use a three-edged needle or plum-blossom needles to tap the affected areas, causing little bleeding, then apply cupping. Treatment is given once or twice a day.

C. Ear Acupuncture

Main points: Neurogate (Ear Shenmen), Adrenal, Subcortex, Occiput.

Method: Select two or three points for each treatment.

Moderate or strong stimulation is used, or the needles are retained for thirty to sixty minutes.

Remarks

Needles must be completely sterilized before application to avoid infection. If ulceration, septicimia and pyemia due to erysipelas-complicated infection appear, combined Chinese and Western measures of treatment should be taken.

52. Urticaria

Urticaria, a common allergic condition, is also known as nettle rash. Most acute cases may be cured completely a short time after attack, but chronic cases, marked by repeated attacks, last months or years.

Etiology and Pathology

Urticaria is caused by collection of pathogenic wind in the superficial layer of the muscles or accumulation of heat in the stomach and intestines that is not removed from inside or outside and settles in the pores of the skin. Sometimes it is also induced by intake of fish and shrimp or by parasites.

Differentiation

Urticaria is marked by the transient appearance of smooth, slightly elevated patches that are redder or paler than the surrounding skin and is often attended by severe inching or sometimes by abdominal pain upon attack; recurrences are frequent in chronic cases.

Treatment

A. Body Acupuncture

Method: Main points are in the Hand-Yangming and Foot-Taiyin meridians. Needling is given with the reducing method, or cutaneous acupuncture is employed.

Prescription: Hegu (LI 4), Quchi (LI 11), Xuehai (Sp 10), Weizhong (B 40), Geshu (B 17), Tianjing (TE 10).

Explanation: Since it is due to exogenous wind attacking the superficial layer of the muscles, Hegu (LI 4) and Quchi (LI 11) of the Hand-Yangming Meridian and Xuehai (Sp 10) of the Foot-Taiyin Meridian are used to eleminate wind and heat through readjusting the qi in the two meridians. Weizhong (B 40), where blood gathers, helps Xuehai (Sp 10) drive away wind and heat from blood. Geshu (B 17), one of the eight influential points dominating blood, combined with Xuehai (Sp 10), treats disorders in the blood. It is especially good for rash red. Tianjing (TE 10), a He (Sea) point of the Triple Energizer Meridian, regulates the burner's function and dispels heat.

B. Ear Acupuncture

Main points: Ear Shenmen, Lung, Occiput, Endocrine, Adrenal.

Method: Needles are retained for fifteen to thirty minutes with intermittent twirling. Treatment is given once a day. Puncture the back of the ear, or prick the posterior auricular vein to induce a little bleeding once a day.

Remarks

(1) Excellent results are seen in treatment of urticaria by acupuncture. It is important to determine the cause of chronic cases and treat the primary affection.

(2) The above treatment can be given to cases of skin inching or dermatitis.

53. Furuncle (Malignant Boil)

Furuncle is a painful nodule formed in the skin, especially in the hand and foot regions. Since when it first appears, it is small but deep rooted, with a hard base like a nail, it is called nail furuncle in traditional Chinese medicine. Different names are given according to the affected areas and shapes. For instance, furuncles occurring on the philtrum are called groove furuncle; those on the fingers are called snake furuncle. If there is a red line spreading upward along the limbs, it is called red thread furuncle.

Etiology and Pathology

Furuncle is usually caused by endogenous toxicity due to extreme heat in the viscera owing to too much greasy food and alcohol. Sometimes it is caused by external affection. When strong pathogenic agents invade the meridians, then attack the internal organs, it is believed a critical condition.

Differentiation

Onset is marked by circumscribed inflammation of the corium and subcutaneous tissue, enclosing a central yellowish of purplish slough, or "core." The root is as hard as a nail. A tingling sensation and slight pain may be present, followed by burning pain and swelling, usually accompanied by chills and fever. If there are high fever, restlessness, dizziness, vomiting, and coma, the toxicity is deep in the interior of the body and septicemia develops.

Treatment

A. Body Acupuncture

Method: Main points are in the Governor Vessel Meridian. Needling is given with the reducing method, or bloodletting is used.

Prescription: Shenzhu (GV 12), Lingtai (GV 10), Hegu (LI 4), Weizhong (B 40)

Explanation: Since the Governor Vessel Meridian governs all the yang meridians, points in the Governor Vessel Meridian are selected. Shenzhu (GV 12) and Lingtai (GV 10) are punctured with the reducing method to eliminate excessive heat in the blood.

These two points are empirical ones in treatment of furuncles. Hegu (LI 4), the Yuan (Source) point of the Hand-Yangming Meridian, which is full of qi and blood, is taken with the reducing method to drive away fire from the Yangming Meridian. It is most helpful to furuncles on the face and lips. Weizhong (B 40), where blood gathers, is used for bloodletting to eliminate heat in the blood.

Modification:

Furuncle in the facial region along the Hand-Yangming Meridian: Shangyang (LI 1) and Quchi (LI 11) are added.

Furuncle on the end of fingers: Quchi (LI 11) and Yingxiang (LI 20) are added.

Furuncle in the facial region along the Foot-Shaoyang Meridian: Yanglingquan (G 34) and Foot-Qiaoyin (G 44) are added.

Furuncle on the fourth and fifth toes: Yanglingquan (G 23) and Tinghui (G 2) are added.

Red thread furuncle: A thick needle is used to prick along the red line until bleeding.

B. Picking Therapy

Method: Find the nodules on either side of the spine, pick them with a thick needle. Treatment is given once a day.

Remarks

In the incipient stage affected areas should not be squeezed by the fingers or picked by needles. It is not advisable to apply puncturing or cupping to the facial area. No surgery is applied to the furuncle when it is red, swollen and hard, to avoid infection. If pus forms, surgery is necessary. Emergency treatment should be given to septicemia.

54. Parotitis (Mumps)

Parotitis is an acute infectious viral disease. It is characterized by redness, swelling, hotness and pain in the parotid region. It often occurs in children in winter and spring. More severe symptoms are found in adults.

Etiology and Pathology

Parotitis is due to affection of epidemic noxious factors and abundant heat in the Shaoyang Meridian, leading to impeded flow of qi. Chills and fever may appear. Since the liver channel is united with the gallbladder in their functional yoke and the Liver Meridian curves around the external genitalia, there is often pain in the swollen testis.

Differentiation

In mild cases symptoms are pain in the parotid region, followed by swelling. If there is no development of other symptoms, the condition will be relieved in several days. In severe cases onset is often accompanied by aversion to cold, fever, headache, vomiting, difficulty in chewing, redness of the swollen parotid region. The most severe cases are manifestated by high fever, restlessness, thirst, swollen testis, superficial, rapid pulse or smooth, rapid pulse, sticky yellow tongue coating.

Treatment

A. Body Acupuncture

Method: Main points are in the Hand-Shaoyang Meridian. Needling is given with the reducing method.

Prescription: Yifeng (TE 17), Waiguan (TE 5), Yemen (TE 2), Jiache (S 6), Hegu (LI 4), Fenglong (S 40), Zusanli (S 36).

Explanation: The affected area pertains to the Hand-Shaoyang Meridian. Yifeng (TE 17), a crossing point of the Hand and Foot Shaoyang meridians, is used to remove obstruction of qi and blood in the local region. The courses of Hand- and Foot-Yangming meridians pass through the cheek region, so Hegu (LI 4) and Jiache (S 6) are taken to eliminate heat. Zusanli (S 36) is used to bring down the heat in the Yangming

Meridian. Fenglong (S 40) is taken to reduce phlegm and fire. Waiguan (TE 5) and Yemen (TE 2), the distal points, readjust the function of the triple burners, clear away heat and relieve swelling and pain.

Modifications:

High fever: Quchi (LI 11) and Waiguan (TE 5) are added.

Swollen testis: Taichong (Liv 3) and Ququan (Liv 8) are added.

B. Ear Acupuncture

Main points: Parotid Gland, Endocrine, Face Area.

Method: Strong stimulation is used. Needles are retained for twenty minutes with intermittent twirling.

Treatment is given once a day when there is inflammation of the testis.

Remarks

Keep the patient isolated until the swelling of the parotid region subsides completely.

Other therapy should be used in combination for severe, complicated cases.

55. Acute Mastitis

Acute mastitis is often seen during postpartum lactation and seldom seen during pregnancy.

Etiology and Pathology

Acute mastitis is usually due to anxiety and irascibility, leading to stagnation of the liver qi or to overintake of greasy food and accumulated heat in the stomach channel, or to affection of pathogenic fire in the broken nipple that obstructs the channels. When the retained milk and fire coagulate, mastitis develops.

Differentiation

The main symptoms are redness, swelling, hotness and pain in the breast, often seen within one mouth after delivery. First, a lump appears in the breast with distending pain, difficulty in lactation, chills and fever, headache, nausea, and thirst. Pus has not yet formed. If enlargement of the breast with redness and burning pain or sometimes with tingling pain appears, it suggests the formation of pus. Acute mastitis is also seen in women in six to seven months pregnancy. At first, the breast skin is normal in colour, but gradually it becomes red and ulcerous. It takes a long time to form pus. The wound will be healed after postpartum.

Treatment

A. Body Acupuncture

Method: Main points are in the Yangming and Jueyin meridians. Needling is given with the reducing method. No moxibustion is used.

Prescription: Zusanli (S 36), Liangqiu (S 34), Qimen (Liv 14), Neiguan (P 6), Jianjing (G 21).

Explanation: The condition is caused by heat accumulated in the Stomach Meridian and depression of the liver. Zusanli (S 36) and Liangqiu (S 34) are used with the reducing method to eliminate heat in the stomach and remove obstruction of the Yangming

Meridian. Qimen (Liv 14) and Neiguan (P 6) are taken to soothe the liver and regulate the qi flow in the chest. Jianjing (G 21), an empirical point for treating acute mastitis, removes the swelling of the breast.

Modification:

Distending sensation due to too much milk in the breast: Shanzhong (CV 17) and Shaoze (SI 1) are added.

Headache and fever: Hegu (LI 4) and Fengchi (G 20) are added.

B. Moxibustion

Method: In the early stages apply a paste of either crushed scallion or garlic to the affected area. Then apply the moxa stick for ten to twenty minutes. Treatment is given once or twice a day.

C. Ear Acupuncture

Main points: Mammary Glands, Endocrine, Adrenal, Chest.

Method: Twirl the inserted needles for some minutes and retain the needles for twenty to thirty minutes.

Remarks

(1) Nipples should be washed clean before and after breast feeding.

(2) Acupuncture therapy is good for the early stages when pus has not formed. Hot compress and massage may be employed to enhance the effect. Surgery is advised for pus-formed cases.

56. Appendicitis

In traditional Chinese medicine this condition is regarded as abscess of the intestines, which is the most common disease in acute abdomen. It is due mostly to obstruction of the appendix cavity or to bacterial infection.

Etiology and Pathology

Appendicitis is usually caused by irregular food intake and imbalance of cold and warmth in the abdomen, or by running immediately after meals. All may disturb the digestive and transport function of the stomach and intestines, giving rise to retardation of qi and blood. Later abundant heat in the intestines meets the stagnated qi and blood, resulting in stale blood and muscles, and abscess develops.

Differentiation

In the early stages pain in the abdomen and umbilicus, then pain moving to the right lower abdomen, fixed pain aggravated by pressure, difficulty in stretching the right leg occur. The symptoms are accompanied by chills and fever, nausea and vomiting, constipation, yellow urine, thin, yellow, sticky tongue coating, rapid, forceful pulse. In cases of severe pain taut abdominal skin or rebounding pain, lumps in the local area, high fever, spontaneous sweating, full, rapid pulse indicate a critical condition.

Treatment

A. Body Acupuncture

Method: Main points are in the Hand and Foot Yangming meridians. Needling is given with the reducing method. Needles are retained for twenty to forty minutes.

Generally, treatment is given once or twice a day. Acupuncture is given every four hours in severe cases.

Prescription: Zusanli (S 36), Lanwei (Extra 33), Quchi (LI 11), Tianshu (S 25).

Explanation: This prescription aims at readjusting the function of the Hand and Foot Yangming meridians, realizing the free flow of qi and blood, regulating yin and yang of the fu organs. In this way the swelling, heat and pain will be relieved. Zusanli (S 36), a He (Sea) point in the Stomach Meridian, is used to promote the Yangming channel's qi. Lanwei (Extra 33) is an effective point for treating appendicitis. It is located in the Stomach Meridian next to Shangjuxu (S 37), an inferior He (Sea) point of the large intestine. Quchi (LI 11) eliminates heat and protects body fluids. Tianshu (S 25), the Front-Mu point of the Large Intestine Meridian, activates the function of the intestines.

B. Ear Acupuncture

Main points: Appendix, Sympathetic Nerve, Large Intestine, Neurogate.

Method: Twirl the needles intermittently and retain them for two to three hours.

C. Point Injection

Main points: Lanwei (Extra 33), tender spots in the abdomen.

Method: A 10 percent glucose solution of 5 to 20 ml is injected into each point. The depth of injection is 0.5 to 0.8 cun. Treatment is given once a day. Distilled water or 5 ml of 0.25 percent procaine solution may also be injected into each point.

Remarks

(1) Acupuncture therapy is relatively effective in treatment of simple acute appendicitis. For severe cases, if there is any possibility of perforation or necrosis of the appendix, surgery is necessary.

(2) For chronic appendicitis, the same points may be used. Treatment is given once a day or every other day. In addition, moxibustion or indirect moxibustion with ginger may be applied.

57. Hemorrhoids

Hemorrhoids refer to varicose dilatation of a vein of the superior or inferior hemorrhoidal plexus, named hemorrhoidal core. This chronic condition is often seen in adults.

Etiology and Pathology

Hemorrhoids are caused by stasis of blood in the anus, attributed to prolonged sitting or walking with burdens on the shoulders, irregular food intake, indulgence of alcohol or spicy food, prolonged dysentery or delivery, general weakness, sinking of qi, mental depression, dysfunction of qi flow, protracted constipation, etc.

Differentiation

Hemorrhoids are internal, external or mixed. Those above or below the anal pectinate line are called internal or external hemorrhoids. Those on the superior and inferior hemorrhoidal plexuses, forming an external and internal hemorrhoid in continuity are called mixed ones. Main symptoms of internal hemorrhoids are bleeding on defecating with bright-red or dark-red blood, prolapse of the pile cores outside of the anus, local severe pain caused by malreduction or inflammation. If inlaid hemorrhoids occur, there may be swelling and distension, erosion, necrosis. Main symptoms of external hermorrhoids are foreign-body sensation in the anus, severe pain or no pain, swelling and pain on inflammation.

Treatment

A. Body Acupuncture

Method: Main points are in the Foot-Taiyang Meridian. Needling is deep, using the reducing method.

Prescription: Ciliao (B 32), Changqiang (GV 1), Huiyang (B 35), Chengshan (B 57), Erbai (Extra 24).

Explanation: Ciliao (B 32), Huiyang (B 35) and Chengshan (B 57), pertaining to the Urinary Bladder Meridian of Foot-Taiyang and its collaterals linking with the anus, are punctured deeply with the reducing method to activate the qi flow in the Urinary Bladder Meridian and remove stasis. Changqiang (GV 1) is used to enhance the effect. Erbai (Extra 24) is an empirical point for treating hemorrhoids.

B. Picking Therapy

Method: Find the hemorrhoidal points on both sides of the spinous processes of the seventh thoracic vertebra and the lumbosacral region. Pick one hemorrhoidal point for each treatment. Treatment is given every seven days.

Remarks

Acupuncture therapy may relieve symptoms. Avoid hot, spicy food and keep bowel movements smooth. Radical treatment may need to resort to surgery.

58. Scrofula

Scrofula refers to tuberculous lymphadenitis, commonly called scrofula neck in traditional medicine. It is often found in children and youth.

Etiology and Pathology

Chronic cases are caused by irritation and mental depression, leading to stagnation of the liver qi and generation of fire, which transform the body fluids into phlegm. The phlegm ascends upward and obstructs the channels in the neck area. Sometimes scrofula is due to weakness of the lungs and kidneys, preventing the lung qi from distributing fluids. The phlegm transformed from the collected fluids obstructs the Shaoyang channels. An acute condition is caused by stagnation of qi and blood due to disharmony of the constructive and defensive energy resulting from invasion by exogenous pathogenic wind and heat.

Differentiation

Scrofula often occurs behind the ear and between the neck and nape. It may also appear in the armpit. At first small lumps as large as beans appear; gradually they grow to the size of plums. There is no local redness or hot sensation. The lumps may move.

An acute condition is manifestated by chills and fever, slight local red colour, distending pain. It is considered to be an excess type. A chronic case is often marked by a prolonged course, afternoon fever, dryness of the mouth, anorexia. If the ulcer is difficult to heal after rupturing, the healed wound reopens or the body is emaciated, it suggests a deficiency type.

Treatment

A. Body Acupuncture

Method: Points are selected according to the affected area. Needling is done with the reducing method. Sometimes warm needling, moxibustion or indirect moxibustion with garlic is applied.

Prescriptions:

Scrofula in the neck area: Yifeng (TE 17), Tianjing (TE 10), Foot-Linqi (G 41).

Scrofula in the neck area: Binao (LI 14), Shousanli (LI 10), Daying (S 5).

Scrofula in the armpit: Jianjing (G 21), Shaohai (H 3), Yangfu (G 38).

Explanation: The prescriptions above promote circulation of qi in the channels, regulate qi and blood, remove stasis and wind and heat.

Modification: Bailao (Extra) and Zhoujian (Extra) may be added.

B. Fire Needling

Method: For an unruptured case insert a red-hot needle into the centre of each node. Treatment is given every two or three days.

C. Moxibustion

Main points: (a) Bailao (Extra), Tianjing (G 21).

(b) Zhoujian (Extra) and the vicinity of the affected lymph node.

Method: Apply moxibustion to one of the two groups alternately. Five to seven moxa cones are used for each point. Indirect moxibustion with garlic is applied to the vicinity of the lymph node.

Remarks

If ulceration has already occurred, it is necessary to consider surgery. No needling is allowed for a pustulated lymph node.

59. Thyroid Enlargement

Disorders of the thyroid gland are characterized by swelling, often accompanied by palpitation, tremor of the hands, excessive sweating, etc. They usually occur in young females and include simple goitre and thyroiditis.

Etiology and Pathology

The disease usually results from exasperation and anxiety, leading to stagnation of qi and blood; formation of phlegm from collection of retarded qi, blood stasis and phlegm in the neck cause the appearance of thyroid enlargement. Sometimes it is due to environmental unadaptability or prolonged drinking of "sand water" (heavy water). Depressed qi may turn into fire and cause yin deficiency in the heart, producing palpitation and shortness of breath. In case of yin deficiency in the liver, tremor of the hands will result.

Differentiation

It is marked by swelling of the neck. Sometimes the neck is remarkably enlarged, but there is no sign of taut skin. In some cases there may be accompanying symptoms, such as stuffiness in the chest, tremor of the hands, palpitation, shortness of breath, flushed face, profuse sweating, exophthalmos, restlessness and irascibility, taut, smooth pulse.

Treatment

A. Body Acupuncture

Method: Main points are in the Hand-Shaoyang and Yangming meridians. Needling is done with the half reinforcing, half reducing method.

Prescription: Naohui (TE 13), Hegu (LI 4), Zusanli (S 36), Tiantu (CV 22), Tianding (LI 17), Tianyong (SI 17).

Explanation: Naohui (TE 13), a crossing point of the Hand-Shaoyang and Yangming meridians, is selected to disperse and regulate the qi of the Triple Energizer Meridian and thus remove obstruction. Because both Hand and Foot Yangming meridians run upward to the neck, Hegu (LI 4) and Zusanli (S 36) are used to regulate the qi of the Yangming meridians and cause qi and blood to flow freely. Tiantu (CV 22), Tianding (LI 17) and Tianyong (SI 17) distributed on the neck, are taken as the local points to promote circulation of qi and blood freely. In this way stagnated qi and blood and phlegm can be removed.

B. Ear Acupuncture

Main points: Ear Shenmen, Subcortex, Endocrine, Thyroid Spot in the ear.

Method: Two or three points are selected for one treatment a day. It is most helpful for simple goitre.

In case of thyroidits Heart, Spleen, Brain Point, and Ear Shenmen are added.

Remarks

(1) Iodine medicine should be given to patients suffering from simple goitre during acupuncture treatment to strengthen the curative result.

(2) Surgery should be considered for cases with marked enlargement of the goitre and a feeling of pressure.

(3) Thyroiditis accompanied by high fever, vomiting, delirium, and thin, rapid pulse is considered a critical condition; emergency measures should be taken.

60. Sprain and Stiff Neck

Sprain refers to injuries of the soft tissues, such as skin, muscles, tendons, ligaments, blood vessels, without presence of fracture or dislocation and wounds. Main clinical manifestations are swelling, pain, and motor impairment in the injured areas.

Etiology and Pathology

Sprain is usually caused by vigorous movements, awkward posture of the body, a fall, pulling and twisting of the tendons and muscles on physical exertion, which lead to impairment of the tendons and joints, causing retardation of the meridian qi and stagnation of qi and blood in the injured areas.

Differentiation

Swelling and distending pain due to stagnation of qi and blood, local redness and dark purple spots appear. New injuries are often marked by mild local swelling and pain aggravated by pressure, considered a mild case. Severe redness and swelling in the injured areas and limitation of joint movements are signs of a severe case. Usually there is no obvious swelling in an old injured area, but relapse of swelling and pain are often seen on invasion of pathogenic wind, cold and dampness. Injuries often occur in the shoulder, elbow, wrist, lumbar region, hip, knee and ankle.

Treatment

A. Body Acupuncture

Method: Points in the injured area are mainly selected. Needling is done with the reducing method. Retention of needle and moxibustion or warm needling is used to treat old injuries.

Prescriptions:

Shoulder: Jianyu (SI 15), Jianliao (TE 14), Jianzhen (SI 10).

Elbow: Quchi (LI 11), Shaohai (H 3), Tianjing (TE 10).

Wrist: Yangchi (TE 4), Yangxi (LI 5), Yanggu (SI 5).

Lumbar region: Shenshu (B 23), Yaoyangguan (GV 3), Weizhong (B 40).

Hip region: Huantiao (G 30), Zhibian (B 54), Chengfu (B 36).

Knee joints: Dubi (S 35), Liangqiu (St 34), Xiyangguan (G 33).

Ankle: Jiexi (S 41), Kunlun (B 60), Qiuxu (G 40).

Explanation: Local points in the injured region are usually selected in treatment of sprain. It is helpful to promote circulation of qi and blood, remove obstruction of meridians and enable the injured tissues to be healed. Local and distal points in the diseased meridians may be selected in treatment of severe cases.

B. Pricking Therapy and Cupping

Method: Tap heavily the tenderness in the injured areas with a plum-blossom needle until bleeding, then apply cupping. It is most helpful for newly traumatic injuries with marked hematoma and prolonged blood stasis and invasion of the channels by pathogenic cold.

C. Point Injection

Method: Inject 10 ml of 10 percent glucose or a mixture with 100 mg vitamin B_1 into the tender muscles. If pain radiates in the injured areas, the needling sensation should reach the painful area. Treatment is given once a day or every other day. It is used for acute sprain of the lumbar region.

D. Ear Acupuncture

Main points: Corresponding sensitive spots, Subcortex, Ear Shenmen, Adrenal.

Method: Needling is given with moderate or strong stimulation. Needles are retained for ten to thirty minutes. Treatment is given once a day or every other day. It is used for acute sprains in all parts of the body and it is good for stopping pain.

Remarks

(1) Acupuncture treatment is effective to some extent for sprains, but fractures, dislocations and severance of ligaments should be carefully excluded.

(2) In some cases massage and medication may be applied if necessary.

Stiff Neck

Stiff neck is also termed as injury to the tendons of the neck, usually caused by an awkward posture in sleep or invasion of the nape by pathogenic wind and cold and disharmony of qi in the local meridians.

After getting up in the morning, one usually finds a tugging pain on one side of the nape. Sometimes the pain spreads to the shoulder and upper arm of the affected side, and motor impairment of the neck appears.

Main points are in the Governor Vessel and Foot-Taiyang meridians. Dazhui (GV 14), Tianzhu (B 10), Jianwaishu (SI 14), Xuanzhong (G 29), Houxi (SI 3) are punctured with the reducing method. Moxibustion is applied to dispel cold, stimulate the circulation of blood and cause the muscles and joints to relax. In case of inability to bend forward or backward, Kunlun (B 60) and Lieque (L 7) are added. In case of difficulty in turning the neck, Zhizheng (SI 7) is added to regulate the qi in the Taiyang meridians. Cupping may be applied to the points near the affected areas. Also, Luozhen (Extra 26) may be used alone or in combination with other points.

Remarks

(1) Acupuncture is very effective for stiff neck. Massage and hot compress may be used after acupuncture.

(2) Use properly high pillows. Avoid cold affection and recurrence.

61. Tinnitus, Deafness and Deaf-mutism

Both tinnitus and deafness are symptoms of abnormal sense of hearing. Tinnitus is characterized by subjective ear ringing. Deafness is loss of hearing. Since the causative factors and treatments of both are similar, they are described in the same section.

Etiology and Pathology

Tinnitus and deafness are caused by sudden rage, fright, and upward disturbance of wind and fire in the liver and gallbladder, leading to obstruction of the qi in the Shaoyang Meridian. Sometimes they are due to invasion of the channels by exogenous pathogenic wind, leading to impairment of these orifices, or to deficiency of kidney qi and its failure to ascend and nourish the ear.

Differentiation

(1) Excess syndrome is characterized by sudden deafness caused by some acute diseases or a distended sensation in the ear and continual ear ringing, not alleviated by pressure. In case of upward disturbance of wind fire in the liver and gallbladder, flushed face, thirst, restlessness, irritation and taut pulse often appear. In case of invasion of pathogenic wind, headache due to cold or heat and superficial pulse are frequently seen in clinical practice.

(2) Deficiency syndrome: Deafness is caused by prolonged illness. There is intermittent ear ringing, worse on exertion or alleviated by pressure. Accompanying symptoms are dizziness, low back pain, nocturnal emission, leukorrhea in women, thin, weak pulse.

Treatment

A. Body Acupuncture

Method: Points are mainly selected from the Foot-Shaoyang Meridian and the reducing method is used for excess syndrome. For deficiency syndrome points are selected from the Foot-Shaoyang Meridian and needling is done with the reinforcing method. Small moxa cones may be applied to points in the affected areas.

Prescription: Yifeng (TE 17), Tinghui (G 2), Xiaxi (G 43), Hand-Zhongzhu (TE 3).

Modifications: Hyperactive fire in the liver and gallbladder: Taichong (Liv 3) and Qiuxu (G 40) are added.

Invasion of exogenous pathogenic wind: Waiguan (TE 5) and Hegu (LI 4) are added.

Deficiency in the kidney: Shenshu (B 23) and Guanyuan (CV 4) are added.

Explanation: Both the Foot- and Hand-Shaoyang meridians curve around the preauricular and introauricular region. Hand-Zhongzhu (TE 3), Yifeng (TE 17) of the Hand-Shaoyang Meridian, Tinghui (G 2) and Xiaxi (G 43) of the Foot-Shaoyang Meridian are used in combination to regulate the qi in the Shaoyang channels. This is the basic prescription for this syndrome. In case of hyperactive fire in the liver and gallbladder, Taichong (Liv 3), a Yuan (Source) point of the Liver Meridian, and Qiuxu (G 40), a Yuan point of the Gallbladder Meridian, are used in combination to eliminate fire. This is based on the rule "choosing points on the upper part of the body to treat disorders on the lower" and "the reducing method is for excess syndrome." In cases of invasion of exogenous pathogenic wind, Waiguan (TE 5) and Hegu (LI 4) are chosen to dispel pathogenic factors from the exterior of the body. The kidneys are associated with the ear, so deficiency in the kidneys prevents their essence from reaching the ear. Thus Shenshu (B 23) and Guanyuan (CV 4) are prescribed to adjust and enrich the primary qi of the kidneys and take their essence to the ear. Ear ringing stops and hearing is regained automatically.

B. Point Injection

Main points: Tinggong (SI 19), Yifeng (TE 17), Hand-Wangu (G 12), Qimai (TE 18).

Method: Inject 5 ml of 654-2 solution or 0.2 to 0.5 ml vitamin B_{12} into one of the selected points bilaterally for each treatment. The depth of insertion of the syringe needle is 0.5 to 1 cun.

Remarks

Several factors cause tinnitus and deafness. Acupuncture treatment is more effective in treatment of nervous tinnitus and deafness.

Deaf-mutism

The condition is often caused by febrile diseases or otorrhea in childhood. Acupuncture is more effective in treating patients who have incomplete loss of hearing. The prescription for tinnitus and deafness may be used in this case. Points on the ear may be punctured to some depth. Treatment is given every other day and ten treatments make up a course. The second course begins after an interval of ten days. If audition has improved but with indistinct speech after treatments, Yamen (GV 15), Lianquan (CV 23) and Tongli (H 5) may be selected in coordination. Patients are advised to strengthen speech training.

62. Swelling and Pain of the Eyes and Night Blindness

Swelling and pain of the eyes are the acute symptoms of eye disorders, frequently seen in acute conjunctivitis, pseudomembranous conjunctivitis and epidemic corneal conjunctivitis. They are termed pink eye due to wind heat or prevalent pink eye in traditional Chinese medicine, depending on their manifestations.

Etiology and Pathology

The condition is often due to affection of exogenous pathogenic wind and heat, which is collected in the body and unable to disperse, or due to upward disturbance of hyperactive fire of the liver and gallbladder along their meridians, resulting in obstruction of the meridian and retardation of qi and blood.

Differentiation

Redness, swelling and pain in the eyes, photophobia, lacrimation, difficulty in opening the eyes may occur. If they are accompanied by headache, fever, and superficial, rapid pulse, the cause is believed to be wind and heat. But if they are accompanied by a bitter taste in the mouth, mental restlessness, fever, and taut pulse, the cause is believed to be hyperactive fire of the liver and gallbladder.

Treatment

A. Body Acupuncture

Method: Points are mainly selected from the Hand-Yangming and Foot-Jueyin meridians. Needling is given with the reducing method.

Prescription: Taiyang (Extra 2), Hegu (LI 4), Shangxing (GV 23).

Explanation: This prescription is used to clear out wind heat, reduce swelling and stop pain. The eye is believed to be the orifice of the liver. The Yangming, Shaoyang and Taiyang meridians meet at the ocular region. Therefore Hegu (LI 4) is used to regulate the qi in the Yangming Meridian and dispel wind and heat. Taichong (Liv 3) is used to activate the flow of qi in the Jueyin Meridian, thus lowering the hyperactive fire of the liver. Jingming (B 1), the point where the urinary bladder and stomach meridians meet, is taken to eliminate accumulated heat in the diseased area. Pricking Shangxing (GV 23) and Taiyang (Extra 2) to cause bleeding dispels heat and reduces swelling.

Modifications:

Disorder due to wind and heat: Shaoshang (L 11) is added.

Disorder due to hyperactive fire of the liver and gallbladder: Xingjian (Liv 2) and Xiaxi (G 43) are added.

B. Pricking Therapy

Method: Find the sensitive spots in the scapular region, the area 0.5 cun lateral to Dazhui (GV 14), or the region of the frontal branches of the superficial temporal artery, midway between the medial ends of the two eyebrows and upper eyelids, then prick the selected spots with a three-edged needle.

C. Ear Acupuncture

Main points: Eye, Eye 1, Eye 2, Liver.

Conjunctivitis may be treated by pricking the ear apex and retroauricular vein to cause bleeding.

Remarks

Needles must be strictly sterilized. Needling is done slowly and gently without lifting and thrusting to avoid infections and bleeding.

Night Blindness

Night blindness refers to blurred vision at night yet normal vision in daytime. It is due to exhaustion of the kidney yin, resulting in inability of the essence to flow upwards to the eyes.

Regulating and tonifying the liver and kidney are taken as the main method of treatment. Ganshu (B 18) and Shenshu (B 23) are punctured with the reinforcing method.

Moxibustion may also be applied. In addition, Xingjian (Liv 2), Jingming (B 1), Guangming (G 37) and Yanglao (SI 6) may be selected in individual cases.

63. Rhinorrhea

Rhinorrhea is manifested by purulent, foul nasal discharge, nasal obstruction, anosmia. It is frequently seen in rhinitis and accessory nasal sinusitis.

Etiology and Pathology

The lung's orifice is the nose. Rhinorrhea is related to invasion of the lung channel by pathogenic factors. When wind cold attacks and accumulates in the body, it may turn into heat, resulting in failure of the lung to disperse its qi and upward disturbance of the nose by the retained pathogenic factors. Finally nasal obstruction appears. If the accumulated heat has not been cleared out after the pathogenic wind is dispelled, it may lead to formation of turbid nasal discharge, blocking the nose, thus causing rhinorrhea.

Differentiation

Rhinorrhea is marked by purulent yellow, foul nasal discharge, nasal obstruction, and loss of the sense of smell. Accompanying symptoms are cough, insidious frontal headache, rapid pulse, thin, white, sticky tongue coating.

Treatment

A. Body Acupuncture

Method: Points are mainly selected from the meridians of Hand-Taiyin and Yangming. Needling is done with the reducing method.

Prescription: Lieque (L 7), Hegu (LI 4), Yingxing (LI 20), Bitong (Extra), Yintang (Extra 1).

Explanation: Lieque (L 7) is taken to disperse lung qi and dispel pathogenic wind. The meridians of Hand-Taiyin and Yangming are externally and internally related and ascend to both sides of the nose. Hegu (LI 4) and Yingxing (LI 20), therefore, are used to regulate the qi of the Hand-Yangming Meridian and clear away heat in the lung. Yintang (Extra 1) is located in the course of the Conception Vessel Meridian close to the nose. Bitong (Extra) is situated on both sides of the nose. The two points are used to remove nasal obstruction and pathogenic heat.

B. Point Injection

Inject 0.2 to 0.5 ml of compound vitamin B into Yingxing (LI 20) or Hegu (LI 4).

One point is used for each treatment. Treatment is given once every other day.

C. Ear Acupuncture

Main points: Inner Nose, Adrenal, Forehead, Lung.

For allergic patients Ear Asthma and Adrenal are added.

Method: Needles are twirled and retained for twenty to thirty minutes or embedded for one week.

Remarks

Acupuncture treatment is effective for chronic rhinitis but not very helpful for chronic accessory nasal sinusitis, so acupuncture is an auxiliary method in treatment.

64. Epistaxis

Epistaxis refers to nasal bleeding. Occurrence of this disorder is usually related to affection of the lung and stomach.

Etiology and Pathology

The lung qi leads to the nose. The Foot-Yangming Meridian originates in the bridge of the nose. Accumulated wind and heat in the lungs or pathogenic fire in the stomach go upwards to the nose, disrupting blood circulation and causing epistaxis. Traumatic injuries can also cause epistaxis.

Differentiation

Nasal bleeding accompanied by fever, cough, etc, is due to heat in the Lung Meridian. Nasal bleeding with symptoms of thirst, mental restlessness, fever, and constipation pertains to heat in the stomach channel.

Treatment

Points are mainly selected from the Hand-Yangming and Governor Vessel meridians. Needling is done with the reducing method.

Prescription: Hegu (LI 4) and Shangxing (GV 23).

Explanation: The meridians of Hand-Yangming and Hand-Taiyin are united externally and internally in their functional yoke and connected with the meridian of Foot-Yangming. Hegu (LI 4) is used to clear out heat from the channels and stop nasal bleeding. The Governor Vessel Meridian is the sea of the yang meridians and hyperactive heat pertaining to yang in the yang meridians will force blood to circulate perversely. Therefore, Shangxing (GV 23) is chosen to dispel heat from the Governor Vessel Meridian and check nasal bleeding.

Modifications:

Heat in the lung: Shaoshang (L 11) is added.

Heat in the stomach: Neiting (S 44) is added.

Continuous nasal bleeding due to traumatic injuries: Finger needling may be used. Kunlun (B 60) and Taixi (K 3) are bilaterally pinched with the index tinger and thumb.

Remarks

(1) Cold compress may be given simultaneously during treatment.

(2) Epistaxis may be seen in various diseases, such as blood disease, vicarious menstruation, infectious diseases and hypertension. Especially, the possibility of tumours

in the nasopharyngeal region should be checked. It is necessary to have consultations and combine methods of treatment in individual cases.

65. Toothache

Toothache is a frequent symptom in oral disorders. Its onset is mainly related to heat accumulated in the stomach channel and deficiency of yin in the kidneys.

Etiology and Pathology

The meridians of Hand- and Foot-Yangming enter the upper and lower gums separately. If there is heat in the large intestine and stomach or pathogenic wind invades channels and accumulates in them, it may turn into fire, leading to upward inflaming of the channels; thus toothache occurs. The kidneys dominate the bones of which the teeth are a part. Insufficient kidney yin may result in fire going upwards and toothache. Overeating of sweet and sour food, uncleaned teeth and mouth or a decayed tooth are also causes of toothache.

Differentiation

Toothache is manifested by foul breath, yellow tongue coating, constipation and full pulse, thus abundant fire in the Yangming meridian. Severe toothache with gingival swelling, accompanied by chills, fever, superficial and rapid pulse, is diagnosed as toothache due to wind and fire. If toothache is insidious, accompanied by thin pulse and loosened teeth without foul breathing, it is due to deficiency in the kidneys.

Treatment

A. Body Acupuncture

Method: Main points are in the Hand- and Foot-Yangming meridians. Needling is given with the reducing method. Distal points on the left may be selected for disorders on the right and vice versa.

Prescription: Hegu (LI 4), Jiache (S 6), Neiting (S 44), Xiaguan (S 7).

Toothache due to wind and fire: Waiguan (TE 5), Fengchi (G 20).

Toothache due to yin deficiency: Taixi (K 3), Xingjian (Liv 2).

Explanation: Hegu (LI 4) is chosen to eliminate heat in the Hand-Yangming Meridian. Jiache (S 6), Neiting (S 44) and Xiaguan (S 7) are used to disperse the qi in the Foot-Yangming Meridian. Waiguan (TE 5) and Fengchi (G 20) are taken to eliminate wind and heat. Taixi (K 3) is used to strengthen kidney yin and Xingjian (Liv 2) to reduce fire in the liver. These two points are prescribed for toothache due to yin deficiency.

B. Ear Acupuncture

Main points: Upper Jaw, Lower Jaw, Ear Apex, Ear Shenmen.

Method: Strong stimulation is given. Needles are retained for twenty to thirty minutes.

Remarks

(1) Toothache should be differentiated from trigeminal neuralgia.

(2) In general, acupuncture is effective for toothache, and it is good for temporarily stopping pain in a decayed tooth.

(3) Observe oral hygiene.

66. Swelling and Pain in the Throat

Swelling and pain in the throat include acute pharyngitis, tonsillitis and chronic pharyngitis. Symptoms of chronic tonsillitis are similar to the above; the same treatment may be given.

Etiology and Pathology

The pharynx is connected to the esophagus and leads to the stomach. The throat joins the respiratory tract and leads to the lungs. If there is abundant wind and fire in the lungs or upwards disturbance of accumulated heat in the lung and stomach meridians, swelling and pain in the throat occur. The condition is diagnosed as an excess syndrome. Depletion of the kidney yin results in inability of fluids to moisten the throat and upwards inflaming, causing swelling and pain in the throat, considered a deficiency syndrome.

Differentiation

Heat-excess syndrome is manifested by congestion and swelling of the throat with burning sensation, severe pain, difficulty in swallowing. If symptoms of cough, thirst, constipation, intermittent headache due to cold or heat appear, the condition is considered affection of the lungs and stomach by exogenous pathogenic wind heat or abundant heat.

Yin-deficiency syndrome is marked by mild congestion, swelling, pain in the throat or pain in swallowing, and mild fever, becoming worse at night.

Treatment

A. Body Acupuncture

a. Heat-excess syndrome

Method: Points are mainly selected from the Hand-Taiyin, Yangming and Foot-meridians. Needling is done with the reducing method.

Prescription: Shaoshang (L 11), Chize (L 5), Hegu (LI 4), Xiangu (S 43), Guanchong (TE 1).

Explanation: This prescription treats any kind of swelling and pain in the throat pertaining to heat syndrome. Shaoshang (L 11), the Jing (Well) point of the Hand-Taiyin Meridian, is a main point in treating disorders of the throat by pricking it until bleeding. It is good for dispelling heat from the lungs. Chize (L 5), the He (Sea) point in the Hand-Taiyin Meridian, is prescribed for abundant heat in the Lung Meridian. Hegu (LI 4) and Xiangu (S 43), pertaining to Hand- and Foot-Yangming meridians respectively, are chosen to eliminate heat accumulated in the Yangming meridians. Guanchong (TE 1), the Jing (Well) point of the Triple Energizer Meridian, may be pricked to cause bleeding to dispel heat from the lungs and stomach, thus reducing swelling of the pharynx.

b. Yin deficiency syndrome

Method: Points are mainly selected from the Foot-Shaoyin Meridian. Needling is given with the half reinforcing, half reducing method.

Prescription: Taixi (K 3), Zhaohai (K 6), Yuji (L 10).

Explanation: Taixi (K 3), a Yuan (Source) point of the Foot-Shaoyin Meridian and Zhaohai (K 6), the crossing point of the Foot-Shaoyin and Yangqiao meridians, which pass the throat, are chosen to regulate the qi of the two meridians. Yuji (L 10), the Xing (Spring) point of the Lung Meridian of Hand-Taiyin, is taken to clear the pharynx and eliminate heat in the lungs. The above three points used in combination enable fire due to deficiency to be removed and body fluids preserved. This is helpful for swelling and pain in the throat due to yin dificiency.

B. Ear Acupuncture

Main points: Throat, Heart, Adrenal.

Method: Needles are retained for ten to twenty minutes with intermittent twirling. This is good for chronic tonsillitis. In cases of acute tonsillitis, Tonsil and Helix I-VI may be added instead of Heart and Adrenal. Needles are twirled with strong stimulation for two to three minutes and retained for an hour. Treatment is given once a day.

Remarks

It is advisable to avoid smoking, alcohol, sour and pungent food.

67. Shock

Shock is a condition in many diseases.

Etiology and Pathology

Shock is caused by acute peripheral circulatory failure due to derangement of circulatory control or loss of circulating fluids, resulting from infection, allergy, hemorrhage, burn, profuse sweating, vomiting, diarrhoea, etc. According to the theory of traditional Chinese medicine, it pertains to a collapse type due to big loss of yang qi.

Differentiation

Main manifestations are pallor, cold limbs, profuse sweating, cyanosis, apathy or restlessness, coma, deep, thin, rapid pulse, lowering of blood pressure.

Treatment

A. Body Acupuncture

Method: Treatment aims at reviving the yang for resuscitation. Main points are in the Governor Vessel and Conception Vessel meridians. Generally, strong stimulation is given with intermittent needle twirling. Moxibustion is applied to severe cases.

Prescription: Shuigou (GV 26), Suliao (GV 25), Neiguan (P 6), Zusanli (S 36), Shenque (CV 8), Guanyuan (CV 4)—for moxibustion.

Explanation: Shuigou (GV 26) and Suliao (GV 25) are used to raise blood pressure, excite the respiratory centre and promote yang, for the two points pertain to the Governor Vessel Meridian. Application of moxibustion to Shenjue (CV 8) and Guanyuan (CV 4) can revive yang for resuscitation. Needling Neiguan (P 6) with continuous twirling can promote resuscitation and raise blood pressure.

B. Ear Acupuncture

Main points: Adrenal, Occiput, Heart, Subcortex.

Method: The above points have the effect of promoting resuscitation and raising blood pressure. Strong stimulation may be given and needles are retained for more than half an hour with needles twirled intermittently. After the blood pressure is raised, prolong the interval of needle twirling.

Remarks

Shock is a critical condition. Emergency measures should be taken. For cases due to drowning and electric-current shock, artificial respiration must be used.

68. Hypertension

Etiology and Pathology

Traditional Chinese medicine holds that hypertension is due to disharmony of yin and yang.

Differentiation

(1) Hypertension due to upward flaring of liver fire is manifested by headache, flushed face, congestive eyes, dryness of the mouth, irritability, constipation, red tongue with yellow coating, taut, strong pulse.

(2) Hypertension due to yin deficiency of the liver and kidneys is manifested by vertigo and dizziness, tinnitus, low back pain, weakness of the legs, palpitation, insomnia, red tongue, taut, rapid pulse.

In either case, if there is evidence of damp phlegm, symptoms of fullness and distress in the chest, palpitation, numbness of the limbs, possible obesity, red tongue, and taut, smooth pulse may appear.

Treatment

A. Body Acupuncture

Method: Treatment aims at pacifying the liver and reducing the fire, strengthening the yin and tranquilizing yang.

Prescription: Quchi (LI 11) and Zusanli (S 36).

Modifications:

Flaring up of liver fire: Taichong (Liv 3) is added with the reducing method.

Yin deficiency of the liver and kidneys: Taixi (K 3) is added with the reinforcing method.

Excessive damp phlegm: Fenglong (S 40) is added with the reducing method.

Headache with distended sensation and dizziness: Fengchi (G 20) and Hegu (LI 4) are added.

Insomnia: Shenmen (H 6) and Sanyinjiao (Sp 6) are added.

Palpitation: Neiguan (P 6) and Xinshu (B 15) are added.

Excessive phlegm: Fenglong (S 40) is added.

Explanation: As Quchi (LI 11) and Zusanli (S 36) are effective in lowering blood pressure, they are chosen as the main points. Taichong (Liv 3) is taken to pacify the liver and reduce fire. Taixi (K 3) is used to replenish the liver and kidneys. Shenmen (H 6) and Sanyinjiao (Sp 6) belong to the Heart and Spleen meridians respectively; they are commonly used to treat insomnia. Neiguan (P 6) and Xinshu (B 15) are used to calm the mind and stop palpitation. These two points also have the function of strengthening the contraction of the myocardium and regulating the rhythm of the heart.

B. Cutaneous Needling

Method: Tap both sides of the spinal column and the lumbosacral region with a plum-blossom needle. The bilateral side of m. sternocleidomastoideus is also used to treat hypertension. The corresponding points on the limbs can be used in combination.

C. Ear Acupuncture

Main points: Groove (for lowering blood pressure), Hypertension Spot.

Method: Treatment is given daily. Ten to fifteen treatments make up a course. Needle-embedding or tip-bleeding technique is used too.

D. Point Injection

Main points: 1) Zusanli (S 36), Neiguan (P 6).

2) Hegu (LI 4), Sanyinjiao (Sp 6).

3) Taichong (Liv 3), Quchi (LI 11).

Method: The three groups of points can be used alternately. Inject 0.5 to 1 ml 0.25 percent procaine hydrochloride into each point daily or 0.1 mg reserpine into each point every other day. Ten treatments make up a course.

Remarks

(1) Acupuncture may render good results in lowering blood pressure.

(2) Vegetables and a low salt and fat diet are good for patients. Avoid stress.

(3) If the blood pressure is measured above 200/120 mmHg, strong stimulation of acupuncture is not allowed.

(4) Renying (S 9) and Shimen (CV 5) are also prescribed to lower blood pressure.

69. Angina Pectoris

Angina pectoris is a paroxysmal thoracic pain, with a feeling of suffocation and impending death, due, most often, to anoxia of the myocardium and precipitated by effort or excitement. It is a main syndrome of coronary heart disease, which is often seen in middle-aged people. The pain may refer to the precordium, left upper arm and left shoulder. It lasts for several minutes and disappears after rest or taking nitrite drugs.

Etiology and Pathology

Angina pectoris is known as true heartache, pectoral pain with cold limbs and pectoral pain with stuffiness in traditional Chinese medicine. It is believed to be caused by obstruction of dampness and phlegm and stagnation of qi and blood due to hyperactivity of the yang in the chest.

Treatment

A. Body Acupuncture

Method: Treatment aims at strengthening the free flow of qi and blood circulation and stopping pain. Points from the Hand-Jueyin Meridian and Back-Shu points are selected. Needling is given with the reducing method. Needles are retained with twirling intermittently.

Prescription: Neiguan (P 6), Jianshi (P 5), Ximen (P 4), Xinshu (B 15), Jueyinshu (B 14), Jiaji points (T_{3-7}).

Explanation: Piercing technique is used on the points on the upper limbs, e.g. needling Neiguan (P 6) towards Waiguan (TE 5), Jianshi (P 5) towards Zhigou (TE 6), to conduct the needle sensation to the elbow and shoulder regions. Clinically, it is proved that Neiguan (P 6) and Jueyinshu (B 14) decrease attacks of angina pectoris and alleviate symptoms. When the Back-Shu points are punctured, the tip of the needle should be inserted obliquely towards the posterior midline. One or two pairs of Jiaji points are selected for each treatment. When the acupuncture sensation appears, the patient may feel the heart being lifted.

B. Point Injection

Main points: Neiguan (P 6), Ximen (P 5), Xinshu (B 15), Jueyinshu (B 14).

Method: Inject 0.5 to 1 ml *Radix Salviae Mitiorrhizae*, compound *Salviae Mifirrhizar* solution or *Radix Ilicis* solution into each point. One or two points are used for each treatment. Points may be used alternately. Treatment is given once a day or every other day. Ten to fifteen treatments make up a course.

C. Ear Acupuncture

Main points: Tender spots of the heart region, Sympathetic Nerve, Subcortex.

Method: Retain needles for fifteen to thirty minutes, or embed needles at the sensitive spots.

Remarks

Acupuncture treatment is good to some extent for angina pectoris. If sharp, continuous pain and cold sweat appear and there is no response to rest, acupuncture or nitroglycerin put under the tongue, there may be myocardial infarction. In this case other treatment should be given.

70. Thromboangiitis Obliterans

This is an inflammatory and obliterative disease of the blood vessels of the limbs, primarily the lower limbs, occurring chiefly in young men and leading to ischemia of tissues and gangrene.

Etiology and Pathology

The disease is usually caused by spasm of blood vessels, leading to retardation of qi and blood, and meridians obstructed because of cold, dampness, toxic and other pathogenic factors. At the advanced stage ischemia of tissues and gangrene may occur.

Differentiation

In the early stages there is insufficient blood in one of the lower limbs with cold sensation, numbness, pale or purple skin of the leg. One may feel a distending pain and spasm in the leg when walking, which is relieved after rest, yet returns upon walking again. Further, there are muscular atrophy and persistent pain, which worsen at night. In the late stages the skin of the limb ends becomes dark, necrotic or scaling. Other symptoms are attenuation or disappearance of the arteriopalmus in the dorsum, posterior tibia and femur, aversion to cold, flabby tongue with thin white coating.

Treatment

A. Body Acupuncture

Method: Treatment aims at activating blood circulation, relieving pain, relaxing tendons and removing obstruction in meridians and collaterals. Needling is given with the reducing method. Needles are retained and moxibustion applied.

Main points in lower limbs: Yanglinquan (G 34), Yinlingquan (Sp 9), Zusanli (S 36), Sanyinjiao (Sp 6), Xuanzhong (G 39).

Secondary points: Weizhong (B 40), Xuehai (Sp 10), Chengshan (B 57), Kunlun (B 60), Taixi (K 3), Chongyang (S 42), Taichong (Liv 3).

Upper limbs: Quchi (LI 11), Neiguan (P 6), Hegu (LI 4).

Explanation: As the disorder often occurs in the lower limbs, points there are mostly selected. If the trouble is in the lateral side of the foot and dorsum, Yanglingquan (G 34), Zusanli (S 36), etc., are taken. If the disorder is in the medial side, Yinlingquan (Sp 9) and Sanyinjiao (Sp 6) are used. Weizhong (B 40) and Xuehai (Sp 10) can activate blood circulation and remove stasis, while Fuliu (K 7), Xuanzhong (G 39), Chengshan (B 57) and Kunlun (B 60) are taken to relax the tendons and activate joint movement. Taixi (K 3), Chongyang (S 41), Taichong (Liv 3) are all closely related to blood vessels; they are the Yuan (Source) points of the kidney, stomach, and liver meridians respectively and can be used too.

If the disorder is in the upper limbs, Quchi (LI 11), Neiguan (P 6), and Hegu (LI 4) can be selected to activate the circulation of qi and blood of the affected limb. Besides, Neiguan (P 6) and Zusanli (S 36) can improve functional activities of the human body.

B. Electroacupuncture

It is good for troubles in the lower limbs. For selection of points refer to body acupuncture. Two or three points are taken for each treatment. Treatment is given once every other day. The current is on for twenty to thirty minutes. Ten to fifteen treatments make up a course.

C. Point Injection

Main points: Xinshu (B 15), Geshu (B 17), Yanglingquan (G 34), Sanyinjiao (Sp 6), Xuanzhong (G 39).

Method: Select two points for each treatment. Inject 0.5 ml of 5 percent Chinese angelica solution or 50 mg vitamin B_1 into each point. Treatment is given daily. Ten treatments make up a course.

Remarks

(1) Keep constantly warm. The affected limbs should do appropriate exercises and avoid traumatic injury to keep away infection and ulceration. Give up smoking.

(2) Acupuncture activates blood circulation and relieves pain. In cases of infection or necrosis surgery should be considered.

71. Urinary-Tract Infection

Urinary-tract infection refers to infection of the urethra, urinary bladder, ureter and renal pelvis.

Etiology and Pathology

Traditional Chinese medicine holds that pathogenic damp and heat in the lower burner results in water metabolic disturbance in the kidney and urinary bladder, leading to abnormal urination. Before long, when dampness impairs yang and the heat consumes the body fluids, the condition may become severe or mild and relapse appears.

Differentiation

(1) Acute case: The condition mostly pertains to a damp heat-type. Clinical manifestations are fever, low back pain, frequency of urination, pain, urgency of micturition on urinating, red tongue with sticky yellow coating, taut and rapid or smooth and rapid pulse.

(2) Chronic case: An acute case that fails respond to treatment. Kidney yin insufficiency is the main reason. Clinical symptoms are lumbago, general lassitude, dizziness, tinnitus, frequency and urgency of urination, mild fever, slight edema, red tongue with thin yellow coating, thin, taut pulse.

Treatment

A. Body Acupuncture

Method: Main points are in the Conception Vessel Meridian and meridians of Foot-Taiyin to clear out heat and dampness. Needling is done with the reducing method in acute cases. For chronic cases treatment is to nourish yin and tonify the kidney with the reinforcing method.

Prescription:

(1) Zhongji (CV 3), Ciliao (B 32), Yinlingquan (Sp 9).

(2) Shenshu (B 23), Sanyinjiao (Sp 6), Taixi (K 3).

Modifications:

Edema: Shuifen (CV 9) and Fuliu (K 7) are added.

Fever: Dazhui (GV 14) and Waiguan (TE 5) are added.

Explanation: The first group of points is taken for acute cases, the second for chronic cases. Zhongji (CV 3), Ciliao (B 32) and Yinlingquan (Sp 9) can be used to clear out dampness and heat in the lower burner and promote urination, while Shenshu (B 23), Sanyinjiao (Sp 6) and Taixi (K 3) are taken to nourish yin and tonify the kidney. Needling Shenshu (B 23) may improve the urinary function of the kidney in patients with nephritis. Shuifen (B 23) and Fuliu (K 7) are the key points for edema, while Dazhui (GV 14) and Waiguan (TE 5) are for febrile diseases. For acute cases with fever, strong reducing method is applied to clear off pathogenic heat.

B. Ear Acupuncture

Main points: Kidney, Urinary Bladder, Occiput, Adrenal.

Method: Select two or three points for each treatment. Needles are retained for twenty to thirty minutes and twirled one or two times. The points mentioned above are more effective in treatment of cystitis. For pyelonephritis, Liver and Endocrine are added.

Remarks

Women should pay attention to hygiene of the vulva in the menstrual period. Change diapers frequently for babies to prevent infection of the urethra.

72. Acute Lumbar Sprain

Etiology and Pathology

Acute lumbar sprain is usually caused by stagnation of blood and traction of muscles and ligaments in the lower back area by force or an awkward posture of the lumbar region on exertion.

Differentiation

Clinical manifestations are sudden lower back pain, limited extension and flexion, local tenderness, swelling, pain radiating to the lower limbs.

Treatment

A. Body Acupuncture

Method: Treatment aims at easing the tendons, activating blood circulation and stopping pain. Main points are in the Foot-Taiyang Meridian, combined with points in the Hand-Taiyang and Governor Vessel meridians. The reducing method or bloodletting is used with a three-edged needle.

Prescription: Yinmen (B 37), Weizhong (B 40), Shenshu (B 23), Shuigou (GV 26), Houxi (SI 3), Lumbago spots on the back of hands.

Explanation: The Foot-Taiyang meridians pass through the lumbar area. Yinmen (B 37), a distal point, is punctured deeply to strengthen the needling sensation and Weizhong (B 40) is pricked until bleeding to ease the tendons and activate blood circulation. The local point Shenshu (B 23) is used to relieve pain. For strong persons Shuigou (GV 26) or the Lumbago spots on the back of the hands can be punctured; when the needles are retained, ask the patient to move his waist. Shuigou (GV 26) regulates the function of the Du channel and is good for lumbago, neck rigidity, etc. Houxi (TE 3), pertaining to the Hand-Taiyang channel and closely related to the Governor Vessel Meridian is effective in treating acute lower back pain.

B. Cutaneous Needling and Cupping

Tap heavily Weizhong (B 40) and tender areas with a plum-blossom needle until slightly bleeding, followed by cupping.

C. Point Injection

Inject 10 ml of 10 percent glucose solution and/or 100 mg of vitamin B_1 deep into the tender spots. Treatment is given once a day or every other day.

D. Ear Acupuncture

Main points: Lumbosacral vertebrae, Sciatic Nerve and corresponding areas.

Method: Needles are retained for twenty to thirty minutes and twirled once or twice to enhance stimulation. Ask the patient to move his waist in treatment.

Remarks

Rest is necessary for acute cases to relax the lumbar muscles. Keep correct posture during labour and avoid overexertion leading to relapse.

73. Periarthritis of the Shoulder

Etiology and Pathology

The condition is often found in middle-aged people, due to deficiency of qi and blood and local affection of wind and cold or persistent strains. It is mostly seen in females. Modern medicine believes that it is a manifestation of chronic inflammation of joint capsules and tissues around the joints, resulting from some chronic degenerative disease.

Differentiation

In the initial stages there may be pain in one or both shoulders. The pain radiates to the neck and arm regions. Less pain is felt during the day, worsening at night. After getting up in the morning, the patient can alleviate the pain by a slight movement of the affected joints. Turning of the shoulder is limited. The patient cannot carry on routine activities, such as combing hair and dressing. Motor impairment develops when there is adhesion of the affected tissues; this is known as a "frozen" shoulder. In addition to periarthritis of the shoulder, the pain is a symptom of myothenositis in the scapular spine, bursitis below the acromion.

Treatment

A. Body Acupuncture

Method: Treatment aims at warming up the meridians, nourishing blood, activating tendons and relieving pain. Needling is done with the reducing method and deep insertion. Local points are mainly used, or the piercing technique is employed.

Prescription: Jianyu (LI 15) or Jiansanzhen,* Quchi (LI 14), tender spots, Yanglingquan (G 34), Tiaokou (S 38).

Modifications:

Myothenositis in scapular: Jugu (LI 16) and Quyuan (SI 13) are added.

Bursitis below acromion: Jianliao (SJ 14) and Naoshu (SI 10) are added.

B. Point Injection

A 10 percent glucose solution (5 ml) is injected into the tender spots once every other day. Ten treatments make up a course.

C. Cutaneous Needling

Tap the tender spots and the affected area with a plum-blossom needle until bleeding; follow with cupping.

Remarks

(1) It is necessary to distinguish between periarthritis of the shoulder, and TB of shoulder joints.

(2) Those who have motor impairment in the joints should persist in functional exercises. The first step is to make the fingers crawl up a wall or to move the arms forward and backward. The second step is to turn the body around with the hands held together or to raise the hands. The third step is to extend the affected arm and do circular movements. Massage may be applied too.

74. Soft-Tissue Injury in the Knee Region

The knee joint is the largest one in the body, and its structure is quite complicated. Therefore, in addition to pain caused by a morbid state other soft-tissue injuries may lead to pain in the knee joint.

---

*Jiansanzhen means the three points Jianyu (LI 15), Jianqian (located 1 cun above the anterior transverse crease of axilla) and Jianhou (located 1.5 cun above the posterior transverse crease of axilla). A piercing needling technique is used from Jianqian towards Jianhou.

Etiology and Pathology

Soft-tissue injury is usually caused by sprain, contusion, a fall, etc. Ligamenta collateralia and ligamentum cruciatum injuries are often seen clinically.

Differentiation

(1) Ligamenta collateralia injury: Clinically, there is ateralia injury in the lateral aspect. Local pain, limitation of movement, swelling, and tenderness on the superior to the medial condyle of the femur may occur. In diagnosis one hand presses the lateral side of the knee and the other holds the melleolus of the foot and makes it turn inside. Pain in the lateral side shows lateral ligamenta collateralia injury. If the turning can be done easily, it suggests fragmentation. When examination is done in a contrary posture, you may find pain in the medial, showing ligamenta injury or fragmentation.

(2) Ligamentum cruciatum injury may be caused by overextension of the knee joint, simultaneously accompanied by ligamenta collateralia injury in the medial aspect. Posterior ligamentum cruciatum may be caused by overflexion of the knee joint, resulting in swelling and distension of the joints without pain. When it is a fragmentation, in addition to swelling, distension in the joint and severe pain, there may appear tenderness. In diagnosis, ask the patient to sit on a bed and bend his knee joint, forming a 90 degree angle. Both hands firmly hold the malleolus medialis of the tibia and try to push it back and forth. If the malleolus medialis moves forward, it shows anterior ligamentum cruciatum injury. If it moves backward, it shows posterior ligamentum injury.

Treatment

A. Body Acupuncture

Method: Treatment aims at easing the tendons, activating the function of the joints, removing blood stasis and relieving pain. Acupuncture and moxibustion are applied to the tender spots and local points.

Prescription: Tender spots, Xiyan (Extra 32), Weizhong (B 40), Yanglingquan (G 34), Xiyangguan (G 33), Xuehai (Sp 10), Ququan (Liv 8).

Modifications:

Soft-tissue injury in the knee region: Tender spots and local points.

Medial ligamenta collateralia injury: Xuehai (Sp 10) and Quequan (Liv 8).

Lateral ligamenta collateralia injury: Yanglingquan (G 34) and Xiyangguan (G 33).

Ligamentum cruciatum injury: Xiyan (Extra 32), Weizhong (B 40), Liangqiu (S 34), Femur-Futu (S 32). Warming needling can be applied to each point.

B. Cupping

After normal acupuncture cupping is given to points such as Xiyan (Extra 32).

C. Point Injection

Inject 1 ml of Chinese angelica compound solution or 5 ml of 10 percent glucose solution into each point near the joint. Avoid injecting the drug into the joint cavity. Treatment is given daily or every other day.

Remarks

See Number 32. "Obstruction Syndromes" for treatment of disorders of the joints. Slight pain in the joints without local abnormal signs and progressive aggravation is mostly due to nervous dysfunction. The above treatment may be referred to and distal points along the channel can be taken.

75. Neurasthenia

Neurasthenia commonly occurs in the young.

Etiology and Pathology

The cause is believed to be long-standing mental stress or poor health after prolonged illness. It is usually related to dysfunction of the heart, liver, spleen and kidney. A deficiency syndrome is often found clinically.

Differentiation

Generally, onset of the disease is gradual. Common symptoms are insomnia, dizziness, headache, tinnitus, poor memory, general lassitude, listlessness, excitation during the night and inability to fall asleep.

(1) Neurasthenia due to deficiency in the heart and spleen: Clinical manifestations are insomnia, dream-disturbed sleep, palpitation, poor memory, pallor, poor appitite, pale tongue, thin, feeble pulse.

(2) Neurasthenia due to insufficiency in the heart and kidney: Clinical manifestations are dizziness, tinnitus, aversion to cold, lumbar pain, frequent urination, nocturnal emission, impotence, deep, thin pulse.

Treatment

A. Body Acupuncture

Method: Points in the Shaoyin meridians and related Back-Shu points are selected to soothe the mind. Needling is done with moderate stimulation. For deficiency of kidney yang, moxibustion follows acupuncture.

Prescription: Yiming (Extra 7), Shenmen (H 7), Sanyinjiao (Sp 6).

Modifications:

Deficiency in the heart and spleen: Xinshu (B 15), Pishu (B 20), Neiguan (P 6) and Zusanli (S 36) are added.

Insufficiency in the heart and kidney: Xinshu (B 15), Shenshu (B 23), Guanyuan (CV 4) and Taixi (K 3) are added.

Explanation: Yiming (Extra 7) is taken to ease the mind. Shenmen (H 7) and Sanyinjiao (Sp 6), pertaining to the heart and the spleen meridians respectively, are used to nourish the heart and strengthen the spleen. Moxibustion is applied to Guanyuan (CV 4), Shenshu (B 23) and Zusanli (S 36) to warm up yang. Three to five points are used for each treatment and needles are retained for fifteen to thirty minutes. It has been proved that needle retention or longer (thirty minutes) moxibustion can inhibit the increasing excitment of the nervous system or the higher cerebral cortex.

B. Cutaneous Needling

Tap both sides along the vertebral column, sacral region, eye region, temporal area and the skin around the ankle joint until bleeding.

C. Point Injection

Inject 5 ml of 10 percent glucose solution into Yiming (Extra 7), Neiguan (P 6) and

Zusanli (S 36). A pair of points are used for each treatment. Treatment is given daily or every other day.

D. Ear Acupuncture

Main points: Subcortex, Ear Shenmen, Kidney, Occiput, Heart, Forehead.

Method: Three to five points are taken each time and needles are retained for ten to twenty minutes or embedded for three to nine days.

Remarks

(1) Generally, neurasthenia is a functional disorder and not an organic one, but symptoms similar to neurasthenia may be seen in some organic disorders, therefore, correct diagnosis is necessary.

(2) Help the patients get rid of worries and have full confidence in overcoming the disorder.

76. Glaucoma

Glaucoma is an eye disease caused by an increase in intraocular pressure that produces pathological changes in the optic disk and typical defects in the field of vision.

Etiology and Pathology

Onset of this disease is related to dysfunction of the Liver Meridian. A depressed liver produces abundant fire and wind, which go upward and attack the eyes. Sometimes the disease is caused by hyperactivity of yang of a deficiency nature, resulting from over-fatigue and consumption of essence.

Differentiation

Main symptoms are ophthalmalgia, headache, rainbow vision, hypopsia, accompanied by nausea, vomiting, mydriasis, hardness of the eyeball.

Treatment

A. Body Acupuncture

Method: Treatment aims at calming the liver and restoring visual function. Points selected from the eye area are combined with points of the four limbs. Slight stimulation is given to points in the eye area.

Prescription: Qiuhou (Extra 4), Jingming (B 1), Fengchi (G 20).

Modifications:

Increase of intraocular pressure: Xingjian (Liv 2) and Sanyinjiao (Sp 6) are added.

Headache and ophthalmalgia: Zanzhu (B 2) and Taiyang (Extra 2) are added.

Explanation: Qiuhou (Extra 4) and Jingming (B 1) are prescribed alternately. Fengchi (G 20) is used to bring down the fire in the liver and dispel pathogenic wind. Xingjian (Liv 2) and Sanyinjiao (Sp 6) are taken to lower the intraocular pressure. The local points Zanzhu (B 2) and Taiyang (Extra 2) are selected to treat headache and eye pain. For severe headache prick Zanzhu (B 2) and Taiyang (Extra 2) until bleeding. For nausea and vomiting Neiguan (P 6) and Zusanli (S 36) are selected to harmonize the stomach and bring down the perversive flow of qi. The reducing method is used for points in the limbs. Treatment is given daily. Needles are retained for ten to fifteen minutes. Ten treatments make up a course.

B. Ear Acupuncture

Main points: Eye, Eye_1, Liver, Kidney.

Method: Needles are retained for twenty to thirty minutes. Treatment is given once a day or every other day.

Remarks

(1) Subjective symptoms of this disease often lead to misdiagnosis. Attention should be paid to severe headache and ophthalmalgia as the possible cause of the disease.

(2) Surgery is advised for those whose symptoms cannot be relieved by acupuncture.

77. Retrobulbar Neuritis

This is an inflammation of the nervus opticus axis, caused by meningitis, sinusitis, poisoning, syphilis, other infective diseases and insufficiency of vitamin B_1.

Onset of acute retrobulbar neuritis is abrupt. Impairment of vision or complete blindness may appear quickly; a dull pain is felt when the eyeball is turned; congestive papillae nervi optici or a normal eyeground may appear upon examination of the eyeground.

Onset of a chronic case is gradual. Attenuated vision for far and near sightedness and central dark spots appear. In the early stages, the eyeground is normal, but in later stages the optic papilla on the temporal side becomes pale, known as temporal side atrophy of optic papillae. In traditional Chinese medicine it is called sudden blindness.

Etiology and Pathology

The disease is mostly due to exasperation and agitation, which cause upward flow of perverted liver qi and stagnation of qi and blood and eye failure, or it is due to fright and loss of consciousness, leading to failure of the qi and blood to bring essence to the eyes. Sometimes alcoholic addiction and too much hot, pungent food cause abundant heat and perversive flow of qi and blood, or overanxiety leads to consumption of blood and failure of the essence to go to the eyes. Both conditions result in the disorder.

Differentiation

Acute cases are manifested by sudden impairment of vision or blindness. If caused by rage and injury of the function of the liver, manifestations are headache, an uncomfortable feeling in the eyes, taut, rapid and strong pulse. If due to fright and fear, palpitation, anxiety, mental confusion, thin, rapid pulse appear. If caused by an upward attack of stomach heat, headache, a distending sensation in the eyes, restlessness, thirst, rapid, strong pulse occur.

Treatment

A. Body Acupuncture

Method: Treatment aims at regulating the circulation of qi and blood, removing obstruction from the meridians, pacifying the liver and restoring vision. The half reinforcing, half reducing method is applied to points in the eye region. Needles are slowly inserted 1.5 cun in depth. When a distending sendation occurs, needles are taken out at once and points are pressed to prevent bleeding. The reinforcing method and/or reducing method is used on other points. Needles are retained for ten minutes. Treatment is done every other day.

Prescription: Qiuhou (located midway between the eyeball and junction of lateral quarter and internal three fourths of the infraorbital), Jingming (B 1), Fengchi (G 20), Ganshu (B 18), Shenshu (B 23).

Modifications: Rage and injury of the liver function: Taichong (Liv 3) and Guangming (G 37) are added.

Derangement of qi due to fear and fright: Shenmen (H 7) and Neiguan (P 6) are added.

Upward attack of stomach heat: Neiting (S 44) and Zusanli (S 36) are added.

Explanation: Qiuhou (Extra 4) and Jingming (B 1), both located around the eyeball, are key points in treatment of eyeball disorders. Fengchi (G 20) is a key point in treating disorders of the five senses. They are taken to regulate the flow of qi and blood, remove obstruction from channels and restore vision. As the liver qi flows to the eye and the essence of the kidney ascends to the eye, Ganshu (B 18) and Shenshu (B 23) are used to tonify the kidney and liver and restore vision. Taichong (Liv 3) and Guangming (G 37) have the same effect. Shenmen (H 7) and Neiguan (P 6) are prescribed to calm the mind. Neiting (S 44) and Zusanli (S 36) are used to promote smooth flow of the stomach qi.

Remarks

Acupuncture treatment is helpful to some extent for retrobulbar neuritis, the earlier, the better. Needles should be inserted deeply into Qiuhou (Extra 4) and Jingming (UB 1). In some cases needles are inserted 2 cun deep, but the operator must have clinical experience. Effective results can be strengthened when combined therapeutic methods are employed.

78. Myopia

Myopia refers to the error of refraction in which rays of light entering the eye parallel to the optic axis are brought to a focus in front of the retina. It is often due to inadequate light during working or reading. Some cases are congenital.

Etiology and Pathology

The eye is believed to be the window of the liver and the essence of the zang-fu organs. If the function of the zang-fu organs is impaired, deficiency of the liver qi may appear and the eyes may fail to see far objects. Sometimes myopia is due to weakness of the heart qi leading to deficiency of yang and abundance of yin. Finally the eyesight is impaired.

Differentiation

Myopia occurs mostly in the young, marked by blurring of vision for far objects or unclear vision in reading. There are no other marked symptoms.

Treatment

A. Body Acupuncture

Method: Treatment aims at strengthening the function of the heart and liver and removing obstruction from the meridians. The reinforcing or half reinforcing, half reducing method is applied. Needles are retained for twenty minutes. Treatment is done every other day.

Prescription: Shenmen (H 7), Neiguan (P 6), Xinshu (B 15), Ganshu (B 18), Zusanli (S 36).

Local points:

(1) Sibai (S 2), Jingming (B 1), Yuyao (Extra 3) penetrated towards Zanzhu (B 2).

(2) Fengchi (G 20), Jingming (B 1), Chengqi (S 1).

(3) Yangbai (G 14), Zanzhu (B 2), Sizhukong (TE 23).

(4) Jingming (B 1), Qiuhou (Extra 4).

The four groups of points may be used alternately.

Explanation: Shenmen (H 7), Neiguan (P 6) and Xinshu (B 15) are used to activate the heart qi. Ganshu (B 18) is taken to regulate the liver qi. Zusanli (S 36) is used to strengthen the middle burner and the acquired constitution. The four groups of points around the eyes have the effect of removing obstruction from the channels and restoring normal eyesight.

B. Cutaneous Needling

Tapping region:

(1) Main points: Zhengguang (Extra, located midway between Zanzhu [B 2] and Yuyao [Extra 3], inferior to the margo supraorbitalis) and $Zhengguang_2$ (located midway between Sizhukong [TE 23] and Yugao [Extra 3], inferior to margo infraorbitalis).

Secondary points: Fengchi (G 20), Neiguan (P 6), Dazhui (GV 14).

Method: Twenty to fifty tappings are given within a diameter of 0.5 to 1.2 cm of the points.

(2) Main parts: Nape, eye region (area around the eyes), temporal region.

Method: Three lines of tapping along each side of the cervical vertebra are given. Horizontal tapping or dense tapping is applied to both sides of the first and second cervical vertebra. Three or four circular tappings are given to the eye region of the margo supraorbitalis and margo infraorbitalis. Five or six lines of tapping are done in the shape of a fan from below to above, taking Taiyang (Extra 2) as the centre in the temporal region. Jingming (B 1), Zanzhu (B 2), Sibai (S 2) and Taiyang (Extra 2) should be tapped more than the others.

Light, moderate or heavy tapping is used according to the condition. Generally, moderate tapping is used. Treatment is done every other day. Fifteen treatments make up a course. The second course starts after an interval of two weeks. Current may be applied.

Remarks

(1) Myopia is a common disorder among teenagers. Early acupuncture treatment or plum-blossom needling brings good results. Mild myopia (below 300 diopter) is easy to cure by acupuncture.

(2) Thirty treatments are necessary. Remove eyeglasses when the eyesight is corrected. Further treatment is given to strengthen the results.

(3) Tell patients the importance of protecting their vision and teach them to massage the points around the eyes and Fengchi (G 20) to improve vision.

79. Gastroptosis

Gastroptosis refers to downward displacement of the stomach (including curvatura ventriculi minor).

Etiology and Pathology

The disease is due to sinking of the qi of the middle burner and weakened function of the spleen and stomach. The spleen controls muscles and the transportation and transformation of nutrients, therefore deficiency in the spleen leads to dysfunction of the organ. The loss of lifting ability brings about gastroptosis.

Differentiation

Patients mostly manifest poor health, general lassitude, poor appetite, stiffness, a distended sensation in the epigastrum and abdomen, a traction sensation in the abdomen, a bearing-down sensation after eating or vomiting and belching, loose stool or constipation, which can be alleviated by a prone position, thin, white tongue coating, deep, thin, weak pulse.

Treatment

A. Body Acupuncture

Method: Treatment aims at strengthening the function of the spleen and stomach. Needling is done with the reinforcing method. Generally, deep insertion of needles is necessary. Manipulation—twirling, lifting and thrusting—is usually used. Needles are for more than thirty minutes. Moxibustion may be applied in combination.

Prescriptions:

(1) Zusanli (S 36), Zhongwan (CV 12), Liangmen (S 21), Qihai (CV 6), Tianshu (S 25), Guanyuan (CV 4).

(2) Jiaji points from Ganshu (B 18) to Sanjiaoshu (B 22), Baihui (GV 20).

Explanation: Zhongwan (CV 12), Liangmen (S 21) and Zusanli (S 36) regulate the function of the spleen and stomach in transformation and transportation. Qihai (CV 6) and Guanyuan (CV 4) invigorate qi, restoring the lifting ability of the internal organs. Baihui (GV 20) is a meeting place of the Du channel and yang meridians. The whole body's qi is governed by the Governor Vessel Meridian. The stronger the qi, the greater its lifting ability.

Tianshu (S 25) regulates the function of the stomach and intestines and dispels abdominal distension. Jiaji points activate the function of the zang-fu organs.

B. Point Injection

Main points: Zusanli (S 36), Weishu (B 21), Geshu (B 17).

Method: Inject 1 ml of vitamin B_{12} or 5 percent Chinese angelica solution into each point on both sides. One or two points are taken alternately. Treatment is given daily or every other day. Ten treatments make up a course.

Remarks

There is no radical therapy yet for gastroposis. Through observation of many cases it is certain that acupuncture can relieve or remove symptoms. A long course of treatment may return the stomach to its normal position. It is generally considered that it is more helpful to have needles retained for about an hour, with intermittent twirling. It is advised that the patient rest in bed, avoid overexertion and eat smaller but more frequent meals.

80. Spasm of Esophagus and Cardia

A functional disorder of the nerves and muscles of the esophagus and cardia is caused by persistent spasm. Clinically, the main symptoms are pain below the sternum or pain in the middle and upper abdomen, difficulty in swallowing and regurgitation of food. The illness is known as dysphagia in traditional Chinese medicine.

Etiology and Pathology

Spasm is often due to emotional factors, such as overanxiety and rage, that injure the liver function and lead to perversive flow of the liver qi to the stomach, impeding the digestive function.

Differentiation

In the early stages, when taking a cold drink or feeling anxious, the patient has a sensation of obstruction in the esophagus and a dull or sharp pain radiating to the precordium, neck or upper arms. Associated symptoms are dry mouth, restlessness, stiffness in the chest, and intermittent difficulty in swallowing. In later stages it becomes more difficult to swallow. Regurgitated food is covered with mucus or blood in severe cases.

The tongue coating is light yellow and the pulse is often taut.

Treatment

A. Body Acupuncture

Method: Main points are in the Spleen, Stomach and Conception Vessel meridians to promote the circulation of meridian qi and readjust the function of the stomach. Needling is done with the reducing method and needles are retained for twenty minutes. Treatment is given once or twice a day, or once every other day for late-stage cases.

Prescription: Tonggu (K 20), Shangwan (CV 13), Zhongwan (CV 12), Shanzhong (CV 17), Sanyinjiao (Sp 6), Zusanli (S 36).

Explanation: Tonggu (K 20) and Shangwan (CV 13) resolve phlegm dampness and bring down the perversive flow of the stomach qi. Zhongwan (CV 13) removes retention of food. Shanzhong (CV 17) promotes the smooth flow of qi and removes obstruction. Zusanli (S 36) and Sanyinjiao (Sp 6) regulate the circulation of qi and blood in the spleen and stomach.

B. Ear Acupuncture

Main points: Cardia, Esophagus, Diaphragm, Subcortex.

Method: Generally, strong stimulation is given and needles are retained for twenty to thirty minutes. Twirl the needles every ten minutes. Treatment is given once a day.

Remarks

Spasm of esophagus and cardia may occur separately, known as spasm of esophagus or spasm of cardia. Points and treatment are the same as above. Acupuncture is effective in early stages.

Spasm of cardia in later stages often causes retention of food in the lower part of the esophagus, resulting in its dilatation. Extreme dilatation of the lower part of the esophagus leads to pressure on the internal organs in the thoracic cavity, resulting in dry cough, frequent shortness of breath, cyanosis, hiccups, hoarse voice. In addition to the above-mentioned therapy, it is necessary to make a correct diagnosis and take other treatment measures.

81. Intestinal Obstruction

Intestinal obstruction refers to any hindrance to the passage of intestinal contents. In general there is mechanical ileus and organic ileus. The latter is caused by congenital deformity of the intestinal tract, intestinal inflammation, tumour, adhesion, volvulus, intussusception, ascariasis, etc., while the former is caused by enteroplegia and enterospasm. The disease corresponds to "retention of food," "abdominal pain," and "vomiting feces" in traditional Chinese medicine. The main manifestations are abdominal pain and distension, vomiting and constipation.

Etiology and Pathology

(1) Intestinal obstruction due to accumulation of pathogenic cold is caused by eating too much raw, cold food, leading to accumulation of food in the intestines, impairing their function.

(2) Intestinal obstruction due to retention of food is caused by irregular meals and greasy food.

(3) Intestinal obstruction due to stagnation of heat in the large intestine is caused by affection of heat that enters the body and consumes the body fluids, resulting in dry stool blocking the intestines.

(4) Intestinal obstruction due to disturbance of ascarids is caused by too many ascarids obstructing the intestine.

Differentiation

(1) Accumulation of pathogenic cold is marked by severe abdominal pain, aggravated by pressure, nausea, alleviated by warmth, decrease or disappearance of borborygmus, constipation, pale tongue with thin coating, deep, tight pulse.

(2) Retention of food is manifested by a distended sensation in the epigastrium and abdomen, pain, aggravated by pressure, nausea, vomiting, constipation, vomiting feces in severe cases, red tongue with sticky yellow coating, smooth or deep, strong pulse.

(3) Symptoms of stagnation of heat in the intestine are distended pain in the abdomen, aggravated by pressure, fever, preference for cold, constipation, red tongue with dry yellow coating, rapid, strong pulse.

(4) Disturbance of ascarids: Severe pain in the abdomen, aggravated by pressure, nausea and vomiting, constipation, intestinal shape seen on the surface of the abdomen, movable lumps, uriticaria all over the body, pale tongue with sticky white coating, taut pulse.

Treatment

A. Body Acupuncture

Method: Treatment aims at removing obstruction and relieving pain. Needling is given with the reducing method and twirling, lifting and thrusting. Moderate or strong stimulations are applied. Needles are not retained in the abdominal points, but for the rest of the points, needles are retained for thirty minutes. Needles are twirled, lifted and thrust for five minutes after an interval of ten minutes. For cases due to accumulation of cold, warming needling or box moxibustion is used for five to ten minutes for each point.

Prescription: Dachangshu (B 25), Xiaochangshu (B 27), Tianshu (S 25), Guanyuan (CV 4), Zusanli (S 36), Shangjuxu (S 37), Xiajuxu (S 39).

Modifications:

Accumulation of cold: Neiguan (P 6) is added.

Retention of food: Zhongwan (CV 12) is added.

Stagnation of heat: Quchi (LI 11) is added.

Disturbance of ascarids: Sifeng (Extra 29, located at the palmar surface in the transverse crease of proximal interphalangeal joints of the index, middle, ring and little fingers) is added and pricked with a three-edged needle until bleeding, and Baichongke, located 1 cun above Xuehai (Sp 10), is added.

Explanation:

Since the trouble is in the large and small intestines, Dachangshu (B 25), Xiaochangshu (B 27), Tianshu (S 25) and Guanyuan (CV 4) are selected, following the principle of combining Back-Shu and Front-Mu points so as to adjust the transporting function of the intestines. Zusanli (S 36) is taken to strengthen the function of the stomach and intestines, promote the circulation of blood and relieve pain. Shangjuxu (S 37) and Xiajuxu (S 39), the inferior He (Sea) points of the Large and Small Intestinal meridians respectively, treat disorders of the fu organs. Neiguan (P 6) stops vomiting. Zhongwan (CV 12), one of the eight influential points dominating the fu organs, removes retention of food and intestinal obstruction. Quchi (LI 11) reduces heat. Sifeng (Extra 29) and Baichongke (Extra) are key points for eliminating ascarids.

B. Ear Acupuncture

Main points: Large Intestine, Small Intestine, Lower Abdomen, Sanjiao, Diaphram, Subcortex.

Method: Strong stimulation is employed. Needles are retained for thirty to sixty minutes. Twirl the needles every five to ten minutes.

Remarks

Intestinal obstruction is a critical condition. Improper treatment may be dangerous. It is important to make a correct diagnosis and give acupuncture treatment as early as possible. Acupuncture is more effective for mechanical ileus and incomplete intestinal obstruction caused by inflammation, ascarids, volvulus and intussusception.

Generally, symptoms are relieved immediately after acupuncture. Two or three treatments are given daily.

If there is no response after three treatments, surgery should be used.

82. Morning Sickness

Etiology and Pathology

Morning sickness is due mainly to general weakness of the stomach qi and reaction to the development of the fetus.

Differentiation

Nausea and vomiting occur after a pregnancy of one month. Vomiting may take place right after food intake or the sight or smell of food. The accompanying symptoms are fullness in the chest, dizziness, blurring of vision and lassitude.

Treatment

A. Body Acupuncture

Method: The points selected are mainly from the Foot-Yangming and Hand-Jueyin meridians. They can stop vomiting by pacifying the stomach qi. Needling is given with the half reinforcing, half reducing method.

Prescription: Zusanli (S 36), Neiguan (P 6), Shangwan (CV 13).

Explanation: Zusanli (S 36) reduces the perversive flow of the stomach qi. Neiguan (P 6) stops vomiting by easing the chest and fetus. Shangwan (CV 13), a local point, treats fullness in the epigastric region.

B. Ear Acupuncture

Main points: Liver, Stomach, Ear Shenmen, Sympathetic Nerve.

Method: Treatment is given once a day, or needles are embedded for one to five days. Massage the points where needles are embedded to enhance the therapeutic effect.

83. Hysteria

Etiology and Pathology

Hysteria is due to mental disturbance caused by upward invasion of fire resulting from anxiety, frustration or depression.

Differentiation

Symptoms include melancholy without any apparant reason, paraphrenia, suspiciousness, paraphobia, palpitation, irritability, somnolence, etc. Sometimes there is a sudden onset of a suffocating sensation, hiccups, sudden loss of voice, convulsions, taut, thin pulse, and loss of consciousness in severe cases.

Treatment

A. Body Acupuncture

Method: The Front-Mu and Yuan (Source) point of the Heart Meridian are used as the main points to tranquilize the mind. Needling is given with the reducing method.

Prescription: Juque (CV 14), Shenmen (H 7), Sanyinjiao (Sp 6).

Modifications:

Stiffness in the chest: Neiguan (P 6) and Shanzhong (CV 17) are added.

Hiccups: Gongsun (Sp 4) and Tiantu (CV 22) are added.

Aphonia: Tongli (H 5) and Lianquan (CV 23) are added.

Convulsions: Hegu (LI 4) and Taichong (Liv 3) are added.

Loss of Consciousness: Shuigou (GV 26) and Yongquan (K 1) are added.

Explanation: Juque (CV 14) and Shenmen (H 7), the Front-Mu and Yuan (Source) point of the Heart Meridian, combined with Sanyinjiao (Sp 6) of the Spleen Meridian, nourish blood and tranquilize the mind. Neiguan (P 6) and Shanzhong (CV 17) relieve the suffocating sensation. Gongsun (Sp 4) and Tiantu (CV 22) conduct the qi downward to stop hiccups. Tongli (H 5) and Lianquan (CV 23) relieve aphonia. Hegu (LI 4) and Taichong (Liv 3) soothe the liver and stop convulsions. Shuigou (GV 26) and Yongquan (K 1) promote resuscitation.

B. Ear Acupuncture

Main Points: Heart, Kidney, Subcortex, Ear Shenmen, Stomach, Sympathetic Nerve.

Method: Two or three points are selected for each treatment with strong stimulation.

常见病的针灸疗法
涂希　著
*
外文出版社出版
（中国北京百万庄路 24 号）
邮政编码 100037
北京外文印刷厂印刷
中国国际图书贸易总公司发行
（中国北京车公庄西路 35 号）
北京邮政信箱第 399 号　邮政编码 100044
1993 年（16 开）第一版
（英）
ISBN 7－119－01530－3／R・89（外）
04300
14－E－2563S